PRAIS

SAVED I

"There is not enough praise in the world to suppoi̇̇ ̶̶ ̶ ̶.
Saved by Sport. This is a collection of so many amazing journeys of inaiv̶i̶ ̶
who have taken life's hard knocks and used a passion to overcome situations
that some would just roll over and accept. As someone who has also used
sports to overcome both internal and external hardships (running, coaching,
volunteering, etc.), I can say that this book captures the real-life struggles
of everyday people and provides inspiring stories that can be a motivation
to anyone that reads the book. I was inspired by the raw detail that was
provided by all involved. Thank you for such an amazing leap into these
true-life stories."

—**Ryan Chukuske**, Multi-Award-Winning and Amazon Best-Selling
Author of *Bigfoot 200: Because, You Know, Why the #@&% Not*, Writer
for *Eat Clean Run Dirty* magazine and *Ornery Mule Racing*

"The uniqueness of the title and subtitle distills the essence and invokes and
invites a refreshing and supportive perspective about trauma and resilience.
The traumatic and tragic experiences of people that the authors have narrated
and the stories of their recovery through sport and other modalities affirm
the latest findings of neurobiological research: the crucial and fundamental
role of somatic practices in healing from trauma and building resilience. After
each case study, the commentaries the authors add provide the necessary
background information to bring things in an educative context and show
guiding principles at work in recovery."

—**Mukin Mutaal**, BSc, PEng-Certified Energy Manager,
Mindful Based Resilience Trainer and Coach

"*Saved By Sport* is an inspiring read for anyone who has had to regain control
of their lives after going through traumatic experiences and events. It contains
real-life stories, and each one points the way to overcoming and thriving
through the building of resiliency."

—**Lenore Riegel**, Public Relations Attorney and Sports Enthusiast

"In reading the stories in *Saved by Sport*, I was reminded of some of the
inspirational stories I read in the Big Book, the standard primer of AA. The
change in mindset that takes each storyteller across the finish line to discover

a reason for living, a way of living, is nothing short of miraculous. Thank you, Marilyn and Paul, for bringing them to our attention. Several psychotherapy clients come to mind who may find this on a suggested reading list this year."

—Linda Klane, LMFT

"I have never been a sports person. I have no hand–eye coordination. But this book spoke to me in its ability to connect with and be helpful for everyone. I truly enjoyed it."

—Steve Bluestein, Playwright, and Author of *Point of Pines*

"Drs. Gansel and Schienberg's book, *Saved by Sport*, captures the essence of remarkable human resilience. Abilities are uncovered, like Michelangelo's sculptures, using sport as the instrument by which innate strengths, dignity, and humanity appear from within. External 'disabilities' of human beings from around the world are transformed by the lived experience of sport. Bravo!"

—Richard Beck, LCSW, BCD, CGP, FAGPA, President, International Association for Group Psychotherapy and Group Processes; Senior Lecturer, Columbia University

"I would like to congratulate both you and Paul for authoring *Saved by Sport*. It is truly an inspiring book filled with short stories and professional commentary about the power of resilience experienced from the insights gained about life through the opportunity of a sport when utilized by a dedicated athlete. There certainly is a unique and obviously powerful mind/body experience charging the life spirit that when tapped into during the action engagement can become truly catalytic and life changing. This is so masterfully evidenced in *Saved by Sport*. I recommend this book to all those seeking inspiration 'from being ordinary to becoming extraordinary' to live their lives."

—Mona Baker, RSMT, RSME, CMA

"*Saved by Sport* is an inspiring book which holds lessons for us all. As we read powerful stories about individuals overcoming often overwhelming physical and mental setbacks through sport and exercise, we can take away positive lessons for our own lives."

—Candace Leeds, Writer, CEO, Candace Leeds & Co.

"*Saved by Sport* is about achievement. It is about individuals who, in a sense, like Horatio Alger, have come back from or conquered a disabling situation. As you read these extraordinary stories, you will be rooting for their courage and resiliency. The beauty of the book is that everyone's story is analyzed from a psychological perspective and explores and uncovers what aided in their successful recoveries. It is exciting, but also a significant learning experience. Well done!"

—**Dick Traum**, PhD, President and Founder of Achilles International

"Many of us look at sports as just a game—a mostly benign way to pass the time or gain a sense of belonging to a team or community. However, as *Saved By Sport* so richly demonstrates, sports can be an avenue for tremendous personal growth and healing—for anyone, at any age. The stories in this book are very personal and incredibly inspirational, and they point the way to a better future for every one of us—if only we'll take the time to follow their example."

—**Peter Economy**, The Leadership Guy on Inc.com

"*Saved by Sport* is about nurturing. Akin to *Hope Dies Last*, Studs Terkel's final inspiring homage to social history in America, Marilyn Gansel, PsyD, and Paul Schienberg, PhD, excel at delivering focused, compassionate, psychological insights by sharing individual stories of restoration, resilience, and yes, hope. You'll discover inspiring stories from ordinary people confronting extraordinary life circumstances who bravely and willingly open themselves to psychological and physical salvation by nurturing and embracing their vulnerability through recreation and the joy of movement."

—**Tim Bayley**, DO, PhD, Chief Medical Officer and Chairman at MedWrite International, http://www.medwriteinternational.com

"Doctors Marilyn Gansel and Paul Schienberg magnificently provide a much-needed practical and inspirational guide for overcoming ANY difficulty one faces in life, resulting in skyrocketing their health, happiness, and success! Each success story strikes a chord in all of us. This is a MUST READ for anyone who has not yet released the giant that resides within!"

—**Jack Singer**, PhD, Performance Acceleration Coach

"Doctors Marilyn Gansel and Paul Schienberg beautifully capture the pure essence of sport and its incredible healing properties through these magnificent stories. The emotional and physical challenges eloquently shared remind us all that participation in sport can truly be 'life saving' and 'life altering.' This inspirational book is a must read for all."

—**Joanne McCallie**, Author of *Secret Warrior: A Coach & Fighter, On and Off the Court*, Former Head Coach of the Duke University Women's Basketball Team

Saved by Sport: True Stories of Ordinary People Facing Extraordinary Hardships; Finding Their Resilient Inner Athlete

by Marilyn Gansel, PsyD and Paul Schienberg, PhD

© Copyright 2022 Marilyn Gansel, PsyD and Paul Schienberg, PhD

ISBN 978-1-64663-577-1

Published by

◄ köehlerbooks™

3705 Shore Drive
Virginia Beach, VA 23455
800-435-4811
www.koehlerbooks.com

A portion of the proceeds will be donated to Special Olympics Florida.

TRUE STORIES OF ORDINARY PEOPLE FACING
EXTRAORDINARY HARDSHIPS

SAVED BY SPORT

FINDING THEIR RESILIENT INNER ATHLETE

With a Foreword by:
Coach P–Joanne P. McCallie, Author of
Secret Warrior: A Coach & Fighter, On and Off the Court

MARILYN GANSEL, PsyD
PAUL SCHIENBERG, PhD

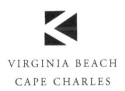

VIRGINIA BEACH
CAPE CHARLES

DEDICATIONS

I dedicate this book
To all those ordinary people facing extraordinary hardships ~ Finding
their resilient inner athlete.
Marilyn Gansel, PsyD

This book is dedicated to my loving parents, Charlotte and Barney. Their
loving support and sacrifices allowed me to grow from a birth defect infant
into a child, and then into an adult who could function normally and
believe I belonged in this world.
So, this book is one part of my "paying it forward."
Paul Schienberg, PhD

TABLE OF CONTENTS:

You Are Stronger Than You Think!

FOREWORD

SPORTS SHAPE LIVES. FOR all of us who have participated in the athletic arena, there are no shortages of lessons, experiences, and opportunities to grow in all ways. In *Saved By Sport*, the authors share compelling and heartfelt stories through detailed narratives that shock the reader while compelling them to find out more with every descriptive word.

Whether it is Lena, Carol, or any of the others, the details and their respective journeys are stunningly adverse. So many tragic and traumatic lives left to cope with events outside of their control makes the reader step back in the wonderment of the cruelty of life's unpredictable nature. The strength, energy, and mental fortitude to seek out sport under the direst circumstances is overwhelmingly courageous and reminds us all of the possibilities of life beyond circumstance and control.

Whether through an "escape" mentality or driving through challenges with a strong faith, the stories reflect a relentless pursuit of sorting through chaos to seek an emotional and productive balance in life. This collection of narratives inspires us directly while reminding us, very profoundly and poignantly, that sport can alter our sense of emotional and physical being forever. We can exist by our choices rather than chance circumstances. We can move past the unthinkable to a place of balance, productivity, and peace in our daily lives.

The power of exercise in creating energy both physically and mentally has been documented in many writings and studies. The body's reaction to such activity is clear. *Saved By Sport* takes the concept of exercise and sport participation to a new and very authentic level. The moving stories, marked by tremendous fortitude and grit, leave the reader with a profound sense of admiration and inspiration with each word and story. We all need to encourage ourselves to find our way to the best physical and emotional balance. *Saved by Sport* is a wonderful collection of writing, filled with the message of hope and action under the most adverse circumstances. The depth of each message and story will no doubt change the lives of individuals. The reading of the book will not only inspire but also honor the storytellers, as they found a way to thrive.

Joanne P. McCallie

Author of *Secret Warrior: A Coach & Fighter, On and Off the Court* and *Choice Not Chance: Rules for Building a Fierce Competitor*

NOTE FROM THE AUTHORS

Disclaimer: We thank all our interviewees for allowing us to share their stories. Each person told their story to us documenting their trauma and how sport changed their lives for the better. We, as the authors, have provided a commentary after each narrative. We also thank author Meg Meeker for her insightful book Strong Fathers, Strong Daughters: 10 Secrets Every Father Should Know. We believe it is a must read for all fathers.

"If there is no struggle, there is no progress."
—Frederick Douglass[1]

ATHLETES KNOW ABOUT MENTAL rehearsal, visualization, confidence, and self-talk. They know these are powerful strength-building tools for winning and reaching their personal best or excellence.

Athletes know they must believe it to become it. They have learned how to deal with stress because they have played their game physically, mentally, and spiritually. And they understand the importance of the mental practice; it is not enough to physically play well. The mind must actively work just as hard as the body.

Athletes have the will to win; they have faced their fears and created a level of self-confidence so they can go out and challenge their opponents

---

1 Frederick Douglass, Frederick Douglass: *Selected Speeches and Writings by Frederick Douglass.*

head-on. Athletes say over and over what they need to hear to be a confident, positive person. While they may have some anxiety before a game, they can "talk" themselves into believing a successful outcome. They know what to do; it has become second nature to them.

We know the true meaning of courage, endurance, empowerment, and resiliency. We are not who we were. Our old stories have changed; they have evolved and will continue to mature. We have found the opportunities and the possibilities from our fights; a new discovery of what we are meant to do and who we are meant to be has developed through our involvement with sport, fitness, exercise, and psychology. Other individuals in this book chose to confront their difficulties using different physical and mental coping mechanisms; but we all have progressed.

AUTHOR'S NOTE BY PAUL SCHIENBERG, PhD

Dr. Marilyn Gansel has been on a similar journey to mine. From the time we met on Marilyn's radio show, our connection was clearly immediate and deep. We learned that we were both interested in interviewing other people who had faced significant challenges and used sport and exercise as the method of healing, overcoming, and building a life that was meaningful and successful. We have compiled their stories in this book, thankful for their willingness to share their tales with us. We hope this book will inspire those who are facing mountains and want to become fit to climb them as we did, through the everyday miracles of sport and exercise.

AUTHOR'S NOTE BY MARILYN GANSEL, PsyD

I personally know that if I hadn't explored the connection between the mind and body, if I hadn't expanded my knowledge of sport, fitness, and psychology, I would not have come full circle to understand myself and others better. I wouldn't know first-hand what makes people strong, more resilient, more able to cope with the inevitable stresses of daily life, and unexpected obstacles that appear immovable. Because of my relationship with life battles, I could give others a chance to experiment with physical and psychological tools to challenge the mindset—and change obstacles into opportunities!

Dr. Paul Schienberg, a Clinical Psychologist, and I feel compelled to share stories of real people and how they used physical, mental, and athletic training techniques to overcome life's hurdles. We feel blessed to share their stories, for they, like us, drew on their life lessons to create flexible systems to survive and prosper like the athletes we have come to admire.

This book is a practical guide for people to develop the necessary tools *to keep going* while facing tremendous adversity. Take resiliency tests; learn how resilient you are now.

Explore with us and experiment with the tools to *train* yourself to think like an athlete so you can perform better if faced with a life challenge. Read our piece on the "10 Ways to Become More Resilient." Share these stories and inspire others to find the courage to change. And, if you prefer to work with us privately, in small groups, or through online workshops, feel free to contact us by email at drpaul47@gmail.com or marilyn@positiveperformancecoach.org to schedule a time to discuss your need.

Both Dr. Paul and I hope that, in reading and understanding these life-changing stories, you will reach the top of your game in life, rebounding with the mindset, resiliency, and tenacity of an athlete.

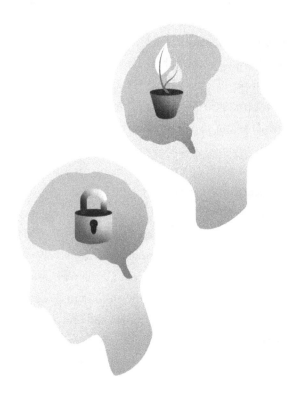

Fixed and Growth Mindsets

PART I

THE MINDSET

CHAPTER 1

WHY MINDSET MATTERS FOR YOUR SUCCESS

COULD WHAT YOU BELIEVE about yourself impact your success or failure? Your beliefs play a pivotal role in what you want and whether you achieve it. It is your mindset that plays a significant role in determining achievement, success, life satisfaction, and fulfilling relationships. So, what exactly is mindset?

A mindset refers to whether you believe qualities such as intelligence, talents, and resilience are fixed or changeable traits. There are two different types of mindsets: 1) People with a fixed mindset believe that these qualities are inborn, fixed, and unchangeable. 2) Those with a growth mindset, on the other hand, believe that these abilities can be developed and strengthened by way of commitment, hard work, and being with people who believe in you and are willing and able to show you a positive direction.

MINDSET FORMATION

Young people are trained in the two types of mindsets from a young age, by parents, teachers, friends, and counselors. Certain characteristics can get assigned to either a fixed or growth mindset.

Fixed Mindsets: Young people who are taught that they should look smart instead of loving learning tend to develop a fixed mindset. They become more concerned with how they are being judged and fear that they might not live up to expectations.

Growth Mindsets: Youngsters who are taught to explore, embrace new experiences, and enjoy challenges are more likely to develop a growth mindset. Rather than seeing mistakes as setbacks, they are willing to try new things and make errors all in the name of learning and achieving potential. The growth mindset is about living up to one's potential. The effort that goes into learning and deepening their understanding and talents is well worth all the toil and trouble.

THE IMPACT OF MINDSET

Your mindset plays a critical role in how you cope with life's challenges. In school, it can mean greater achievement and increased effort. When facing a problem, such as trying a new job, facing new challenges, people with growth mindsets show greater resilience and success. They are more likely to persevere in the face of setbacks, while those with fixed mindsets are more liable to give up and fall into despair. Growth mindsets, on the other hand, result in hunger for learning. A growth mindset also results in a desire to work hard and discover new things, tackle challenges, and grow as a person. People with a growth mindset who try and fail tend not to view it as a failure or disappointment. Instead, it is a learning experience that can lead to growth and change.

CAN YOU CHANGE YOUR MINDSET?

The answer is simple! YES! It takes certain conditions, however. One of those conditions is to find a mentor, whether it be a teacher, coach, relative, or a friend that cares about you and believes in you. This person can point out the abilities and possibilities that you can't see in yourself. You might not be able to take what they see in you as truth. Stick with it and keep listening to what he or she says. Instead of platitudes like "you are so smart," that person will commend you for your hard work and comment about how you approached the life challenges. They will be more interested in your process in meeting new challenges than your scores on tests. This kind of input will improve your confidence in taking on all of life's experiences. Your mindset will change from fixed to growth.

CHAPTER 2

LENA'S STORY: BIKES, BLADES, PILATES KO'D MY PTSD

"The movement of my body during sports allowed me to release the great amount of rage inside me. After playing, I could always think more clearly."

I GRADUALLY BECAME MORE conscious and aware of my troubling situation. Then, around my adolescence, it surfaced. It was as a teenager that I really started seeing things.

I grew up in a very challenging home situation, where my parents only seemed to get along. From when I was one year old to about ten, you would have been able to look on ours as a normal family, with the usual few problems here and there.

My grandparents, who were Italian, were anxious to get their children settled, so my mother married my father when she was seventeen. She had me when she was eighteen. It was an arranged marriage. They didn't go on one single date before saying, "I do." My father was eight years older than my mother.

I JUST CLEANED THE BLOOD OFF AND SAT BACK DOWN.

My father was handsome and my mother very beautiful, and at the beginning, their marriage had some positives. Things started to change when I was about eleven or twelve. There were a lot of fights, screaming matches. My mother became prone to bouts of depression and panic. Sometimes she would go straight to bed after my father went to work, leaving me with my sister and my brother, both younger. So, I assumed the role of the caretaker. Sometimes I would call my grandfather and let him know that my mother had taken to her bed again, that she had another panic attack because she was so unhappy with my father. When she had these attacks, it was like she died and went away.

When I realized that both my parents were terribly unhappy, it became necessary that I become the caretaker of the family.

My father started having more explosive bouts in arguments with my mother, now including threats of violence. He said things like, "I'm going to kill you." He would shout this threat to my mother, brother, sister, and me, at the same time letting us know he had a gun in the garage. "I'll shoot you all in the middle of the night." I became hypervigilant because of these threats. My house felt like a war zone.

I developed PTSD, because whenever my father came home, the arguments would get explosive. He'd throw dishes and take knives out of the drawer and get very violent with me and my brothers and sister. I remember my father telling my brother that he was a jerk, he was a donkey, and he would never amount to anything. My mother would cringe, but she would never take a stand against him. So, I stood up to him, telling him he had no right to say that to my brother. My father's response was to lean across the table and slap my face. I felt a crunch in my nose, and blood was dripping down my face. I just went to the bathroom and cleaned myself off.

Then I kept on eating to show him that he was not going to get to me.

SPORTS, THE HEALTHIEST ESCAPE ROUTES

My father had become a monster, and I became the protector, as my brothers and sister were petrified. I didn't want to stay home, because the fighting there continued. I had to develop a persona of strength, becoming hyper-involved in doing things that strengthened me and allowed me to feel like I existed. Exercising made me feel less depressed and gave me a sense of myself, so I got a bicycle and rode it every day. I started roller blading. I learned yoga on my own. In high school, I took trampoline and track and field. There was something about doing those things that kind of saved my life, because they got me into the world.

Exercise helped me become aware of my body. It made me feel grounded in the world. This was my defense. Maybe it was a crazy defense, but it worked. My father was a bully, but I was going to fight back. I was not only fighting for me, but I was also fighting for my whole family. My mother couldn't leave because she was a good Italian Catholic who didn't believe in divorce, which would bring shame on the family.

Not even my grandparents stood up to my father. I was always saying to them, "Are you all crazy? Don't you understand that he's terrorizing us? Don't you know my mother is getting sicker and sicker? He's not healthy. He's terrorizing us with violence. My brother John is getting more depressed!" And they still didn't understand, so I chose the healthiest ways for me to escape.

I was also active in school. I had mentors who had no idea what was happening in my home and who acknowledged my work. They would actually ask me to talk to other kids who were having a hard time at school, but I never let my mentors know that things were unraveling in my own life. To all appearances, I was the perfect person, the student everyone liked. I had the best personality.

But when I went home, I still had to protect myself, my siblings, and my mother who always wanted to know why I was so active. Why I was in so many clubs. What was wrong with me? She wanted me home, probably to protect her. Why was I doing yoga?

At about this time, my father confronted me with weird personal attacks about how stupid I was, about how ugly I looked. He told me that my mother was raising a child that was out of control. What is the expression? The pot calling the kettle black! So, I bought myself a yoga book, and that's when I was downstairs at fourteen, doing yoga by myself, including the advanced poses that would gain me strength. These were the things that kept me going. I kept saying to myself that I'm not going to have a life like they had. I'm going to survive.

One day, I was sitting in front of my neighbor's house talking to my friend, Pat, who had invited some boys in the neighborhood to come over to join us. We were just sitting and talking, that's all. My father called me into the house, but I didn't go right away. He called me again. Then he called me again, and I went home. As I walked in the door, he grabbed a shoe—a wooden clog shoe—and smashed me over the head with it. I felt a crack and blood pouring out of my head, and I started screaming.

BRINGING THE ABUSE HOME TO MY HEART

My mother was not in the house. He rushed me up the steps, grabbed me, and told me that I couldn't tell anyone. I said, "What are you, crazy? What are you doing to me? Are you trying to kill me?" It's like a scene from *Carrie*. He took me to the doctor but made me swear that I would not admit what had occurred. I got stitches in my head, and had to tell my mother, grandparents, my brother, and my sister the same lie. They were skeptical but were too afraid to say anything. They protected themselves. It remained a secret for three years.

The verbal and physical abuse and threats continued and even got worse.

I responded to all this craziness by continuing to be active in all the sports, as well as joining the modern dance club. I also wrote, directed, and acted in a play for the kids in my neighborhood. It was about vampires, and I was so proud of it. At that time of my life, I was into *Dark Shadows*. At the end of the performance, what did my mother do? She took me upstairs and said, "How dare you humiliate me with that nonsense in front of people. You are such a fucking idiot!" and slapped me in the face. I was too much for her. She found me unbearable because I was defying my father, and they were always fighting about me. She was sick of me.

Again, my response to this latest assault was to take classes in art and ballet, which I paid for by getting a part-time job at a pharmacy. I was fourteen years old at the time.

I know it's hard to imagine, but my father got even more abusive. So, in order to focus on my homework, I had to move into the basement. He would follow me downstairs to taunt me, and I would do my best to ignore him.

I learned to put up a protective shield as he kept hammering at my appearance. One day, I was walking in front of my parents, and I heard my father saying to my mother, "Look at her. Look at the way she walks. She has an ugly walk. Isn't she disgusting?" My mother said nothing.

One time, we were at a wedding, and when a guy asked me to dance, my father cut in and grabbed me, telling the guy to get lost. His was grinding his teeth as he growled to me, "If you go out with a guy, I will kill you. I will step on you until your guts come out of your mouth."

Despite my protests, I internalized much of what my father said and began to think badly about the way I looked. My exercising became not so much about being healthy and strong, but a way for me to become thin and attractive.

When I lost ten pounds during high school, people started to ask if I was okay. No, I wasn't. I was becoming very weak and had to go to the school psychologist who was also very concerned about me. I told her about my home situation, and her advice was to leave my home as soon as possible. This was not very helpful, since I had nowhere to go. Then I found a woman therapist I liked a lot, and she became a role model. She had a bicycle out in her yard and would bike to her job. I wanted to be like her, to be athletic and help people.

My eating got better, and I got stronger. But I still had an image of myself as damaged.

Now I was more the geek with thick glasses, always reading and singing in the choir.

Around the same time, things got worse in my family. My sister, who was now fourteen years old and the real pretty one, started using heroin and decompensating. I tried to intervene, asking her to change her behavior and sharing my concerns, but she pushed me away like most drug users do. Her friends told her they thought I was weird, a goody two shoes. She tried to turn me into a bad girl and set me up with hoodlums. I wouldn't go for it, though.

AFTER MOVING MY BODY, I THINK MORE CLEARLY

One day, I went over to my sister's boyfriend's house. He was a drug user, as was a friend of his who was there. I never used, but I tried to help him by becoming his caretaker, which was for me another way of surviving, while my sister's way of surviving was to numb herself out.

The physical activities I was doing helped me develop a positive relationship with my body, but at the same time, my sister kept getting worse. I went out with the guy I was trying to help for about three years, until I finally had to let go of that situation in order to move forward.

I graduated from high school, despite all the stressors in my family and the relationship I ended. I went onto college, even though the message from my parents was that a woman's role is in the home. While I was going to college, I started seeing a therapist at the Washington Square Institute who helped me make the break from my family and leave home. It was not easy. I watched my brother have a nervous breakdown and get hospitalized, which forced him to drop out of flying school, his lifelong dream. He has since been diagnosed as a schizophrenic.

I feel like the only true survivor of my family situation. I have been living a real life.

My sister is still around. My brother is still around and living with my mother. They have a total codependent relationship. My father died four years ago, after my mother had secured a divorce from him.

I had to work through a lot of things to get to a place where I feel I have a right to survive. I focused on committing to my education, graduate work, improving my mental health with psychotherapy, and sports.

I did a Pilates training program, am training to be a Pilates teacher, and hope to be certified soon. I entered Queens College, where I loved the classes and students, and was very active and engaged with so many of the creative people there.

Of course, I continued with my bike riding, rollerblading, and dance. I majored in education and minored in psychology and art. After college graduation, when I moved out of my house, I remained out of contact with my family for about one year, knowing they would have tried to drag me back home and back to my caretaker role.

I chose life instead of death.

Today, I am also helped by art therapy, a nonverbal means of communicating, very similar to movement therapy in that it allows someone to express feelings and thoughts without words. It helped identify the feelings that had long been rumbling around inside me.

The movement of my body during sports allowed me to release the great amount of rage inside me. After playing, I could always think more clearly. People are often surprised with what comes out during these nonverbal forms of therapy, the considerable relief that you feel when a powerful emotion is no longer bottled up, but out in the open. Things go from unconscious to a conscious place, giving you awareness, so you can begin to work on your issues.

Through these many modalities, I've come to a place where I don't have to always take care of everybody, where I can allow someone to be there for me. My husband has a background in movement therapy, and he also used this form of treatment to better connect with himself.

We've been together for twenty years. It took a long time to meet the right guy for me. All the other men I allowed into my life were there to find something deficient in me. But he never cared about those things.

When I met him, I knew I was finally at home.

COMMENTARY BY MARILYN GANSEL, PsyD

"A daughter needs a loving, available, predictable father or father figure who can be counted on, whether divorced or at home. She needs his best paternal intentions, even if his efforts occasionally fall short. She needs his maturity and limit setting and sexual oppositeness, so that she can function with confidence in the wider world of adult love and work."

—Victoria Secunda [2]

FROM THE MOMENT THE child sees and feels her father's touch or hears his voice, she is in love. A father is a daughter's first love. That attachment, if withheld, if denied, if mistreated can have severe psychological, physical, and emotional consequences that remain with the daughter if not addressed.

Lena shares with us an impactful story of early parental abuse which poignantly affected the way she saw herself, thought about herself and her relationships with others, in particular with young men. She watched her sister's demise into the world of drugs, her brother's nervous breakdown, and her mother's divorce. All this was a result of the abusiveness both verbal and physical that Lena and her family endured for years.

In the book, *Strong Fathers, Strong Daughters*[3], author Meg Meeker states, "Fathers inevitably change the course of their daughters' lives—and can even save them. From the moment you set eyes on her wet-from-the-womb body until she leaves your home, the clock starts ticking. It's the clock that times your hours with her, your opportunities to influence her, to shape her character, and to help her find herself—and to enjoy living." A young girl needs a positive male influence in her life![1]

For Lena, no such father was present. What her father said about her body, for example, created a damaged self-image, poor self-esteem, and a distorted view of her anatomy. Girls, especially at puberty and as young

---

2   Victoria Secunda, *Women and their Fathers: The Sexual and Romantic Impact of the First Man in your life.* Delacorte Press, May 1992.
3   Meg Meeker, MD, *Strong Fathers, Strong Daughters: 10 Secrets Every Father Should Know.* Regnery Publishing, September 5, 2017.

teens, need a role model in a father that is strong, nurturing, and loving; his unequivocal behavior in her life remains very important in shaping her future career, self, and relationships.

In her book, Meeker goes on to share statistics about teenage girls and the traumatic effects a father's negative influence can have on her:

> "Parent connectedness is the number-one factor in preventing girls from engaging in premarital sex and indulging in drugs and alcohol.
>
> - Daughters who perceive that their fathers care a lot about them, who feel connected to their fathers, have significantly fewer suicide attempts and fewer instances of body dissatisfaction, depression, low self-esteem, substance use, and unhealthy weight.
> - Girls with involved fathers are twice as likely to stay in school.
> - A daughter›s self-esteem is best predicted by her father›s physical affection.
> - Girls with a father figure feel more protected, have higher self-esteem, are more likely to attempt college, and are less likely to drop out of college.
> - Girls with fathers who are involved in their lives have higher quantitative and verbal skills and higher intellectual functioning.
> - Girls with good fathers are less likely to flaunt themselves to seek male attention.
> - Fathers help daughters become more competent, more achievement-oriented, and more successful.
> - Girls with involved fathers wait longer to initiate sex and have lower rates of teen pregnancy. Teen girls who live with both parents are three times less likely to lose their virginity before their sixteenth birthdays."

But Lena survived these statistics. She created a world where she could feel confident, empowered, and empathic to the needs of others. She found support through therapy, found a role model with whom she could connect. She sought physical activities that helped her find a positive relationship with her body. She was able to attend school, graduate college, always conscious about improving her mental health with psychotherapy and sports. She found other ways to express her feelings and thoughts, art and movement therapy, and Pilates. She understood the importance of how her energy in sports and therapy could help her work through her problems at home.

In the June 2014 IDEA Fitness Journal, the article "Train Yourself Happy,[4]" by Shirley Archer, JD, MA, gives us reasons why exercise improves mental health. One of the ways exercises enhance mental health is that it increases blood flow and energy; our brain, in the process, gets healthier. Exercise releases emotional stress and boosts self-efficacy as we will see in Matt's story. Exercise can foster social contact since exercise frequently occurs with others. Exercise brings us outdoors where the sunlight and the outside environment helps lift our mood. It certainly diverts negative thinking and encourages engagement instead of avoidance. Exercise teaches persistence.

Lena is an excellent example of how sports and movement and art therapy changed her thinking, and her life, making her story a powerful and inspirational healing force.

---

4   Shirley Archer, JD, MA, "Train Yourself Happy." IDEA Fitness Journal, June 2014.

CHAPTER 3

TRISHA'S STORY: NEVER SURRENDER HERO

TRISHA'S STORY WAS SUPERBLY described by Dr. Paul Kiell, a psychiatrist, runner, and national class swimmer, in his book, *It is the People, a memoir: Stories of the precious unforgettable souls met in the worlds of road running and swimming.*

Dr. Keill has given us permission to share this excerpt from that book (edited for clarity).

Her story follows:

THE CENTRAL PARK JOGGER

Shortly after 9 P.M. on April 19, 1989, in Manhattan's Central Park, twenty-eight-year-old Trisha Meili, associate in the Corporate Finance Department of Salomon Brothers Inc., a Phi Beta Kappa graduate of Wellesley College holding a Yale graduate business/international relations degree, was about to gain an alias, the "Central Park Jogger."

She was rendered unconscious and comatose after being bludgeoned, raped, bound, gagged, and left to die.

Parts of her story, as summarized below, come from personal correspondence and informal conversation. Most, however, is gleaned from portions of her best-selling book, I Am the Central Park Jogger: A Story of Hope and Possibility (New York: Scribner, 2003). The book contains her search for facts about this period, culled from newspaper, hospital, and doctor reports, and from interviews with medical personnel who had treated her. From these accounts she began to learn what had happened, given that she had no recall for the event and for the weeks that followed.

EXTRAORDINARY TRAUMA

Trisha described what happened to her as an "extraordinary trauma." It was, rather, a totally horrendous devastating trauma. This summary will be focusing particularly on the role of exercise in her rehabilitation from extensive brain damage.

Before this night, Trisha had run three Boston Marathons (best time 3:40) and many 10k races. She was determined to run that night (April 19), determination and compulsivity being characteristic features of her makeup. Her last memory, before the run—she entered the park at 84th Street and would run uptown to the poorly lit 102nd Street crossover—was a five-o'clock phone call. Then there is a void in recall until six weeks later.

As she ran along the 102nd Street drive that crossed through the park, she was dragged down into a ravine. Trisha was punched, kicked, raped, hit in the left side of her face with a brick or rock; her eye socket was shattered. Three and a half hours later, unresponsive, bleeding profusely, eye puffed out and almost closed, she was found in a ravine in Central Park lying prone with "airway compromise respirations."

MASSIVE BRAIN DAMAGE

During the ambulance ride to Metropolitan Hospital, the EMTs were unable to get an accurate blood pressure reading. She was hypothermic with a body temperature of eighty-five degrees. There were five deep cuts on her face. Her skull was fractured; her arms and legs were flailing violently, indicative of massive brain damage.

Upon admission to Metropolitan, she was graded on the Glasgow Coma Scale (3-15), a commonly used neurological scale. Fifteen is normal consciousness and brain function; three is totally unresponsive or just being alive. Trisha was graded 4-5 because she did have eye responses.

There was extreme swelling of her brain. "Permanent brain damage seems inevitable," read a portion of the admitting note to Metropolitan Hospital. Her face was unrecognizable to a friend who came to identify her. The attempt to remove a breathing tube eight days later was unsuccessful. She was comatose for twelve days. On the fourteenth day, a memo was sent to employees at Salomon to the effect that she had been removed from the ventilator and could utter single and two-word phrases.

PROGNOSIS: SEVERE COGNITIVE DYSFUNCTION

On May 1, Trisha had begun to awaken from her coma. She began to identify simple words on flash cards, could say "hello" to her father, and could move her eyebrows voluntarily. "She still suffers moments of delusion and fluctuates between lucid and unresponsive," read her chart. Also, she had pneumonia with a temperature of 106 and was "not well oriented to time and place." But on May 9, she was noted to be better oriented to time and place.

Two weeks post-coma, her chart read, ". . . signs of severe cognitive dysfunction suggestive of widespread cerebral impairment . . . at this point she manifests limitations in all areas of cognitive functioning . . . The severity of the patient's condition causes serious concerns about her prospects for long-term recovery. However, it is far too early to make predictions concerning outcome."

Dr. Kurtz, director of the Surgical Intensive Care Unit, had thought she had less than a 50 percent chance of recovering normal brain function. He had told the family that chances for life were 50 percent, and that severe brain damage was likely. Her first clear memory was May 26 when she told a loquacious visitor friend to "shut up."

TREATMENT BEGINS

On June 7, seven weeks after the attack, she arrived at Gaylord Rehabilitation Hospital, a 109-bed non-profit long-term, acute care hospital for adults in the hills of Wallingford, Connecticut. She was then unable to work the buttons on her shirt, unable to walk, unable to remember where to go for therapy sessions. She felt devastated by her failure to remember what she'd read a second ago or think on any but the most rudimentary level.

Her treatment was multi-focused using varied modalities. Not the least of these would be the compassionate approach of the total staff. Exercise was at first focused on relearning balance and how to walk. Then, one fine day in August, she encountered a chapter of the Achilles Track Club at Gaylord.

HER INTRODUCTION TO ACHILLES INTERNATIONAL

Achilles International is a worldwide organization that both organizes and encourages people with all kinds of disabilities—amputation, arthritis, cancer, cerebral palsy, cystic fibrosis, multiple sclerosis, paraplegia, stroke, traumatic brain injury, and visual impairment—to participate in running. Its beginning was in the 1970s, the inspiration of Dr. Richard Traum, himself an amputee. A few words about Traum:

At age twenty-four (in 1964), he was the victim of a freak accident at a gas station where his legs were crushed between two cars. Ultimately the accident would rob him of his right leg, lost to amputation above the knee, and add to his life an interminable time in hospitals for treatment and rehabilitation. But he was still determined to get on with his life. His story, recounted in the following chapter, was one of defeat turned into victory. In 1976, he was the first amputee to complete the NYC Marathon.

TRISHA'S FIRST RUN

For her first run at Gaylord with the Achilles group, she tried to run a hilly quarter-mile loop. She described her initial difficulties with this course, and her final navigation of it, an accomplishment that to her seemed monumental. She wrote:

"And, oh, it felt good! I was acutely aware I was taking back something that belonged to me but had been taken away: the joy of running."

Three months later and seven months after the incident, she walked out of Gaylord, ready to face the world, including a return to full duty at Salomon Brothers.

TRISHA'S INSPIRING NEW PURPOSE

And what of Trisha Meili today? Here, as the late Paul Harvey might put it, is the rest of the story:

In September 1996, she married Jim Schwarz, a Sales consultant (I met him, very nice guy). She left Salomon Brothers in 1998. In a total career change, she became president of The Bridge Fund of New York, Inc., a nonprofit organization whose mission was to prevent homelessness of the working poor who are threatened with the loss of their housing but do not qualify for government assistance.

Trisha continued to work with the Achilles International. After her encounter with the Gaylord Hospital chapter, she had returned to New York and continued to get stronger. She had met with founder Dr. Dick Traum and became an Achilles guide at Saturday workouts in the early 1990s. In 1994, she was Dick Traum's guide in the New York City Marathon.

In 1995, she became a board member and was elected the first chair of Achilles in 2001. In addition, she also became a board member of Gaylord and is now secretary of the board. Finally, she became an advocate trainer of SAVI, Mount Sinai Hospital's Sexual Assault and Violence Intervention Program.

In the spring of 2001, Trisha left The Bridge Fund. Soon after that, she spoke at Spaulding Rehabilitation Hospital about her injury and recovery to a group of physicians, clinicians, brain-injured patients, and families. It was, for Trisha Meili, a profound moment.

It convinced her that she needed to share her story of recovery and healing in a more public way. In the fall of 2001, she began to write her book. Once it was written and published, because of speaking requests from all kinds of organizations, she became a motivational speaker.

HOW RUNNING HELPED HEAL

In a personal communication, Trisha Meili told me that a return to running was a significant contributor to her cognitive recovery. In 1995, she would complete the New York City Marathon in a time of 4:31. "Not too bad!" she wrote in a recent e-mail. Not too bad, indeed! So, too, has been her work in inspiring others who have suffered similar injuries. Some of that work began with a published study where she was both a participant and one of the study's authors. It was research that examined the exercise habits of 240 individuals with traumatic brain injury, comparing the exercisers with the non-exercisers. Those who were active exercisers had fewer overall complaints and symptoms compared with the non-exercisers who, in turn, complained of more cognitive symptoms, suggesting that exercise may improve otherwise diminished cognitive faculties. Also, the exercisers were less depressed. This may indicate a linkage between the emotional and the physical.

The real limitation of the study was that it was retrospective, depending on history, memories, without allowing for other confounding factors that may have determined whether a person chooses to exercise or not. But since then, there have been better studies hinting at the value of exercise in the rehabilitation of people with brain damage from any cause.

WHAT IS KNOWN FROM THESE STUDIES?

Scientists have used sophisticated techniques to measure blood flow to the brain during rest and during exercise. The areas where blood flow seems to seek out and predominate are the hippocampus and its dentate nucleus. They, in turn, are part of the cerebrum. The cerebrum regulates specialized functions such as memory, orientation, perception and judgment, reasoning and thinking. These are the cognitive processes. Their geographic location corresponds to where the teacher says, "Put on your thinking cap." Before describing the studies, a brief orientation to the brain is in order.

BRAIN ANATOMY 101

The brain, unlike other organs such as skin, was always thought to be unable to repair itself, unable to regenerate tissue. Such a conclusion has now been overturned. The area where new memories are laid down, the dentate nucleus, is a region where brain tissue regeneration occurs. The phenomenon of tissue regeneration is termed neurogenesis. To better understand some of the underlying mechanisms, a brief bit of neuroanatomy now may help. The cerebrum or "thinking cap" consists of rounded bundles or lobes. There is the frontal lobe, which, true to its name, is in the front of the head. Just below it, on both sides, are the temporal lobes. They reside at the level of the temples.

The hippocampus is a region in the lower portion of the temporal lobe of the cerebrum. The name derives from its shape, like that of a mythological creature. Its dentate nucleus is embedded in it. It is called dentate because of its tooth-like projections. A nucleus is like a hub, a series of interconnected nerve cells and their fibers (axons). The hippocampus, through its dentate nucleus, is concerned with basic drives, emotions, and the formation of recent memories.

You can liken these higher centers—particularly the dentate nucleus— to a finely tuned Stradivarius violin, delicate and sensitive to changes in climate, humidity, and human tinkering.

You can say, too, that the cerebrum, along with its dentate nucleus sub-region, is a high-maintenance complex. The dentate nucleus, a center sensitive to any of the subtle and not-so-subtle circulatory changes that come with aging, is particularly susceptible to damage and destruction.

THE ADVANTAGE OF INCREASED BLOOD FLOW TO THE BRAIN

Now onto some of the findings that will help explain Trisha Meili's remarkable recovery. In one part of an experiment, exercising animals were determined to have larger blood flow to the dentate nucleus. This increased blood volume coincided with increased findings of neurogenesis.

In the next part of that experiment, eleven exercising humans were instructed to exercise three hours a week for three months. Memory tests were administered at the onset of their exercise regimen. Exercise in the eleven humans, as in the animals, was also found by MRI to have an enhanced effect on blood flow to the dentate nucleus. Furthermore, the increase in blood flow to this area correlated directly with improved scores on memory tests and improvements in overall physical fitness.

The increased blood flow, a by-product of overall fitness, reminds us of the correlation between healthy mind and healthy body. This is an ancient concept, one verbalized in the Roman era when the satirist Juvenal said that our prayers should be for a sane mind in a healthy body (mens sana in corpore sano).

Another study linking heart and blood (cardiovascular) fitness to fitness of brain tissue was conducted in 2006 at the University of Illinois. Here, fifty-nine otherwise healthy but sedentary volunteers, ages sixty through seventy-nine, were randomly assigned to aerobic training or to toning and stretching. For comparison purposes, twenty young adults underwent MRI's, otherwise not participating in the study. Both groups also had MRIs of their brains taken at the beginning and end of the six-month study.

Significant increases in brain volume of the cells and tracts in the brain were found only in the older adults who participated in the aerobic fitness training.

IN CONCLUSION

One can conclude again that fit body equals fit mind. As a result of physical fitness, you can expect to find the heart pumping larger quantities of blood to the brain, the areas that need the "high-octane fuel," specifically the areas that control memory and link to the brain's emotional centers. With these enhanced volumes of blood come the essential fertilizers— oxygen and blood sugar (glucose).

A study from Finland observed that the rates of dementia and Alzheimer's disease among regularly active persons were less than half those among inactive persons. This hints at the promising role for exercise: A vigorous lifestyle may either prevent or retard the dementia of Alzheimer's disease. Short-term memory losses, furthermore, often are the first sign heralding Alzheimer's disease. The first structural breakdown is often in the sensitive dentate nucleus of the hippocampus.

As an aside, there is another culprit terrorizing the dentate nucleus— Type 2 diabetes mellitus. The onset of this malady is usually in middle or later life. Here the blood sugar (glucose) vital to brain function has difficulty getting into tissues and cells.

Studies on humans found that the higher the blood sugar level, the lower the test results for total recall. In other words, where the utilization of blood sugar—the fuel for intellectual function—was impaired, mental functioning was correspondingly impaired. Vigorous exercise, on the other hand, enhances the transport of blood sugar into the cells and tissues.

A STORY OF HOPE AND POSSIBILITY

Trisha Meili's book has a subtitle saying it is a story of Hope and Possibility. So, given the story of her life and the above studies, here are some possibilities.

Whatever can be done to benefit the circulation to the aging hippocampus region of the brain might slow the progression of the various degenerative processes—such as Alzheimer's disease—that assail the aging brain. Similarly, whatever can be done to utilize blood glucose—the brain's principal nutrient—would benefit the hippocampus with its function of recent memory processes.

Enter vigorous exercise with its known ability to enhance blood flow to the brain and to lower blood glucose. Exercise, before the discovery of insulin, was a known treatment for children thought to be pre-diabetic. Exercise encourages glucose utilization in bodily tissues, cells, and organs. Vigorous exercise also increases blood volume and enhances blood flow, carrying with it its vital nutrients of oxygen and glucose to the brain.

Exercise, in a sense, becomes the Viagra of the brain—particularly the aging brain—restoring failing cognitive functions.

Years later, Dr. Robert S. Kurtz told Trisha Meili how amazing it was that her heart was still pumping away. Part of the reason was that she was in ". . . excellent athletic condition—and you're an indomitable person. You were in a situation where other people like you might well be dead—and you weren't."

TRISHA'S WORK FOR CAUSES

Trisha continues to speak and work for noble causes. Her dynamite synergistic alliance with Dr. Richard Traum, founder of Achilles International, has resulted in studies proving the positive benefit of exercise in traumatic brain injury and autism. Among their shared causes is the 'Hope and Possibility Run' that began in 2003. It was after the book by Trisha Meili, I Am the Central Park Jogger: A Story of Hope and Possibility.

Beginning in 2003, with the number of runners in the hundreds, the 16th anniversary race had near 6,000 runners. Earlier, it had become worldwide, and September 2016, saw 3,300 runners from Achilles Mongolia competing in their H&P, the largest among several throughout the world. Achilles Mongolia is only a sample of their membership in seventy-four countries with over 20,000 athletes and volunteers.

Trisha sums up her work and her work with Dick and all the people they have helped along the way:

As it turned out, the attack, meant to take my life, gave me a deeper life, one richer and more meaningful than it might have been.

COMMENTARY BY MARILYN GANSEL, PsyD

I VIVIDLY REMEMBER TURNING on the news that day in 1989 and hearing of the brutal beating and rape of the Central Park Jogger.

In my own head, I wondered how anyone could physically and mentally survive after incurring such savage behavior.

What we learned months later is that traumatic brain injury is not always a death sentence. And Trish, alias the Central Park Jogger, is a testament to "hope is possible." When doctors pronounced her inevitable prognosis—severe cognitive dysfunction—Trisha showed us that her inner, resilient athlete would emerge victorious.

The outpouring of research on brain regeneration that links exercise with increasing brain volume is a huge step for individuals recovering from sexual assault, amnesia, traumatic brain injury, and any neurological impairment. What is also exciting is that studies prove the effectiveness of aerobic exercise for Alzheimer's and Type II Diabetes patients. Just imagine the benefits to our health if we start exercising in our youth and continue that regimen as we mature! Our bodies might be stronger, fitter, and healthier, our minds more confident and focused.

Trisha had been a dedicated runner before her traumatic brain injury. While her recovery was arduous, her ability to choose to regain her courage, strength, and cognitive ability through running is significant.

Even more astounding was the support she received from Achilles International, Dick Traum, and the individuals who challenged and encouraged her to move. Without that community of individuals with physical and mental limitations, she might have not seen such a dramatic recovery from cognitive dysfunction.

PSYCHOLOGICAL COMMENTARY BY DR. PAUL SCHIENBERG

THE TRAUMA THAT TRISH received was remarkable.

It is often the theory that the victim of a trauma gets better quickly if she can remember all the aspects of incident that caused the trauma.

Some treaters push the victim to recall all the details of the incident immediately. Especially with trauma to the head and brain, it is impossible to recall the details. It depends on the part of the brain that is affected by the injuries. Regardless, there is a counter point of view. Sometimes the mind is protecting itself from remembering because the details would just be too overwhelming. It would send the victim into another traumatic experience. The mind often knows what is best. Taking it slowly might, in fact, be the best approach. Take it slow and easy.

At the beginning of Trisha's recovery, she had very little or any memory. In fact, she had lapsed into a coma for a few weeks. It is horrible to think that she might be so injured that she may not come out of the coma. Another way of looking at it is that her brain needed to shut down and not remember what horrible things she had just been through.

When she came out of the coma, her husband was present at her hospital bedside. She was asked many questions by the helping staff of nurses and doctors. Most of the questions had to do with things about the incident that Trish was not able to remember and therefore couldn't answer. Her husband would answer the questions for her. Instead of feeling grateful that he was there to provide the answers, she became very angry with him.

Why? Because she could not answer the questions due to an inability to remember and/or she was not ready to hear what had happened to her. She wanted him to shut up. She would have been psychologically overwhelmed and caused another trauma in talking about what details she could remember. Another reason for her not responding to the questions was that it pointed out that she had lost significant cognitive function, obviously valued in her work life, home life, etc. She would worry if she would ever get those abilities back. She was nowhere near ready to think about that possibility.

Trisha's physical abilities were very important to her. She was an avid runner. After the traumatic incident, she would not be the same athlete. How was she going to deal with that psychologically? She had run alone for years and hours each day. It was a precious ritual in her life. It gave her a great sense of self. Now? Now that she had lost the ability to run as much—and not as fast, if at all—now what? She needed to find a way back to her sport.

She was introduced to Dick Traum, the founder of Achilles International whose focus was to help disabled people get back to participating in sports. Part of their program was to get other disabled athletes to help each other participate in sports. The organization exists in sixty-three countries now. Trish got involved. She saw other disabled people participate in various sports. Many of the participants were even more disabled that Trish. She grew to accept the organization and its mission and regain contact with the sport she loved. She couldn't perform at the high level she did before the traumatic events. But, belonging to a group with similar issues can lead people to accepting a new life—like it did with Trish. She began to accept her new life as a person and an athlete. Achilles International is a powerful medicine for all of us and, for us to believe we do belong and not to collapse. Also, helping others with physical and mental problems can provide courage to go forward. Trish did that and she still is.

CHAPTER 4

CAROL'S STORY: MIRACLES ON MY MAT BY MARILYN GANSEL, PsyD

My Attackers Had Cut the Phone Lines. So, Who Could Rescue Me?

"I am still amazed at how exercise can change whole thought patterns—how movement can help people see life more clearly . . . I now know I can provide hope and healing through Pilates."

THERE I WAS IN my bathroom, blindfolded and gagged, my hands tied behind my back. The gang had left me mercilessly beaten and bleeding, lying on the floor, alone and terrified.

And they might very well return to finish the job.

My attackers had cut the house phone lines. So, who could rescue me? Who would ever find out that I was in the bathroom, hands wired behind my spine? I could smell and taste my own blood. I thought to myself, this is just another injury, just another one for me to withstand.

It appears my life's destiny was a series of "accidents" or "events" that left me in excruciating pain. Would my life be a series of nothing but physical and emotional wounds?

Could I heal from this attack and move on?

THE ACCIDENT THAT SET OFF A CHAIN OF LOSSES

I was born in South Africa, the child of parents who owned and ran a large farm. My siblings and I enjoyed life in the Midlands among the cattle, sheep, chickens, dogs, and horses. We were encouraged to ride and progressively compete in equestrian show jumping.

At the age of twelve, a riding accident left me with my broken neck in a brace and in and out of traction for two years. Unable to play sports with my friends, I became socially isolated; for years, I endured agonizing pain.

I withdrew more and more. I lost everything: my drive, my motivation, my circle of companions, my ability to play sports, my social connection with my friends, and the final straw—my best friend, my horse. My injuries not only caused me physical pain, but also the mental agony of pain that demanded my full attention. Pain consumed me. Not consciously, but subconsciously, I nurtured the torment, which drove me into a spiral of depression. I tried to show a stoic side—strong, impervious to suffering— but other incidents confined me further and contributed to my feelings of discontent and despair.

I barely managed my studies at school. My thinking had become cloudy, and it became difficult for me to absorb information. I lost all motivation to focus. Feeling robbed of joy, I became desperate and suicidal.

There was no one to help me at that time; I was on my own. So, I began a quest to find a purpose—a career that would bring me fulfillment and perhaps ease the emotional and physical burden I experienced every day. I was accepted to a Bible college but didn't finish my studies there. I felt so imprisoned; the teachings of the school—their ideals and beliefs— seemed set in stone. The rigidity of the doctrines drove me to questioning, and I shook the system by asking provocative questions. As a result, I lost faith in the church and its system and left. Still struggling to find a career that would suit me, I began to work at my family business as a receptionist.

Soon, a longing overcame me to find something I could call my own. I decided I wanted to help people through a nursing career, but I quickly learned that this path was not something I could follow. So, I dropped out of nursing school (a pattern?) because I just didn't fit in. I once again questioned their system, their practices, and their disinterest in patients' care and treatment.

For example, I worked on a hospital floor for patients with terminal illnesses, though death was hard for me to deal with. I was told that I could not bring my emotions to the job; I could not become attached to the patients. But I did become attached. I think the last straw was the day I witnessed nurses taking care of a woman who had overdosed on drugs. As the staff was performing CPR to revive her, you could hear her ribs snapping one by one while they laughed and hooted, "So what if she died, she wanted to take her own life anyway!"

WHAT NEXT, I WONDERED?

Luckily, I got an opportunity to work for a large mountain resort as a receptionist. And, this time, I loved my job. It was a perfect fit. I was out in the country enjoying fresh mountain air, glorious sunrises and sunsets, and closeness to Mother Nature—a healer! Even though I was still experiencing physical discomfort, somehow this locale induced serenity of mind, the start of my emotional wound healing. But this idyllic situation would not last long. The resort was undergoing financial difficulties, eventually couldn't afford to pay me, and I had to leave. So, it was back to the family business, this time working myself up the ladder.

Meanwhile, I married a man who was physically abusive. I often wondered if this physical and emotional abuse was what I expected for myself. Did I not think I deserved a better life? Did I attract pain and suffering?

DID I ATTRACT THIS ATTACK TOO?

That's the background to the attack that began my story. Here's what happened.

After my divorce from the abusive husband, I was living on my family farm. On the day in question, our workers were out in the fields. It was lunchtime, and I was alone in my bedroom when I heard noise coming from the kitchen. Five men in blue overalls, like the ones our workers wore in the field, came bursting into my bedroom. They jumped on me, pinning me to the bed.

I tried to call out for help, but the invaders had me in a stranglehold. Blood started pouring out of my nose; I couldn't breathe. I was going to the window with a metal soap dish to break the window open. After slamming the dish against the glass, and breaking it, I squeezed my broken body through and ran to a neighboring farm where I got help.

NIGHTMARES THAT DON'T NEED THE DARK

Most people's nightmares occur at night, but mine were ever present—day and night. In addition to my serious injuries from past accidents and abuses—broken neck, nose, ribs, arm—was this horrific gang attack, which left me with more surgeries and ongoing back and sciatica problems.

I hadn't wanted to see a psychologist, but appointments were made, so I went, not being able to think for myself at this stage. I guess the most beneficial aspect of treatment was learning that during an attack such as this, the brain suddenly remembers the most crucial survival skills. I remembered viewing my body from above and detaching myself from the physical torture. I remembered that no matter what happened to me that day, I remained aware, knowing who I was, at peace. I remembered being grateful that my family was not there to witness or be a part of the attack.

HEALED BY GOD AND PILATES

I found that my healing balm was gratitude. I was grateful to God for not forsaking me and protecting me. I was grateful because there was nowhere else to turn but to the *divine*. I was grateful because He was leading me to the greatest force, and that power was within me. I could make choices—to be still, to listen, and be grateful.

I began to feel life coming back into my bones. I began to feel more clarity, more stability, connecting more with people and with God. I found new strength—power to do what needed to be done.

I knew the only way I could get through everything I endured and heal completely was to move my body again, get the chemistry going. Years of not moving almost destroyed me. I knew whatever exercise I did now would have to be gentle because of my neck and back injuries. I started slowly with simple floor exercises called Pilates, to stabilize my spine.

These movements saved my life! I did basic breathing and postural exercises. They elated me. My pain was no longer as excruciating as in the past. Everything became easier—more focus, better concentration, quality sleeping. I calmed down a lot.

After the gang attack, my nightmares had become frightening reminders of what occurred. I tried concentrating on studying psychology, but suddenly, during exams, I wouldn't be able to remember anything. Apparently, the attack caused stress-related responses and blockages. During this time, I chose to take antidepressants but found the medication didn't really change anything. What did change was my choice of focus—I could concentrate on feeling good or feeling bad. I could choose to be brave or to cower—to give up or not give up.

"THE REMEDY FOR MY PAIN AND SUFFERING WAS EXERCISE."

Just before my mother died, she said, "Carol, you need to know something. Your strongest quality is that you never give up." She told me I was a fighter—that in spite of all the accidents, injuries, and pain I experienced, I could survive and thrive.

Not only did I not give up on this strengthening practice, I became a Pilates instructor. I am still amazed how exercise can change whole thought patterns—how movement can help people see life more clearly. People who need help now gravitate toward me. I am attracting those who need Pilates and relief from pain, whether physical or emotional.

Victory doesn't always last forever. Like an addict spiraling into a hole of despair and depression, I fell again—not literally, but figuratively. A few years ago, I received news that someone close to me had committed suicide.

I was so broken emotionally that I stopped exercising all together. I started smoking and drinking too much, abusing myself. I lost a lot of weight. I was no longer interested in being with people or doing anything. Eventually, a friend I used to take walks with dragged me out of the house, and my healing slowly restored. We started exercising, and soon my mood lifted, and my mind, spirit, and body were revitalized. We always walked in nature since we lived at the beach. That helped me connect with my loved one in spirit. I felt at peace again. The remedy to my pain and suffering was exercise; I knew this would be my panacea, and it was, even after my mother died.

I now know something about the human spirit: We are capable of more than can be imagined. We can forgive unconditionally and offer respect regardless; we can find peace within, no matter what is going on around us. We can expect health when we pursue it, and we can find joy if we choose it.

I now know I can provide hope and healing through Pilates.

COMMENTARY BY MARILYN GANSEL, PsyD

JOSEPH PILATES

Joseph Pilates was a German-born circus performer and boxer who, at the onset of World War I while living in England, was sent to an internment camp where he developed a series of exercises he and others could do on a mat. There, he began to work with detainees rehabilitating them from injuries and illness. Pilates own self-development and interest in the human body and physical prowess of the Greeks along with the practices of Zen and Buddhism further inspired him to invent resistance equipment like the reformer, and the magic circle. Pilates knew that fitness included building body, mind, and spirit. So, while the exercise machines and the mat workout he developed strengthened the body, they also improved the mind and spirit.

THE INTEGRATION OF THE MIND, BODY, AND SPIRIT

Athletes know the power of the mind, body, and spirit. Their practices for their sport depend not only on physical practices but their mental and spiritual thought patterns. They rehearse visualization and mental rehearsal techniques, so when their defenses are down, when a mistake occurs, they call upon their inner athlete to change thought patterns and create more positive ones. This is a process; mental toughness is a set of learned attitudes and tools for athletes to use on their game.

CAROL'S ATTITUDE & GRATITUDE

While Carol was not involved in a team sport, she was deeply committed to her equestrian friends and the joy she entertained when riding. Her equine accident put a sudden end to her pleasure. Just like an athlete who receives a life-changing injury, she experienced isolation, depression, and suicidal thoughts. Carol, who also was abused, recalled the healing power of Mother Nature as well as the immense potential in incorporating gratitude in her life to change negative thought patterns. Gratitude improves physical and mental health. Coupled with her newly found exercise, Pilates, Carol's mind, body, and spirit could deal with adversity, pain, and illness.

PAYING IT FORWARD

We often hear that *when one door closes, another one opens.* When tragedy happens suddenly, it is difficult to perceive that something good comes of it. For Carol, her Pilates discovery led her to a passion for helping and healing others. As a teacher of Pilates, Carol is providing health-building restorative therapy for her students. She is bringing out the inner resiliency and tenacious athlete in the ordinary person.

CHAPTER 5

PAUL'S STORY: EXERCISE EXORCISED MY DEMONS

"I went back to the person I really am—open, honest, thoughtful, considerate, and childlike, mindful and grateful for things."

LIAR!

"You ruined our lives! If I saw a street bum, I would see your face. You shattered our family; we never had a father. You continually broke promises to us. Our trust in you has been broken. You're a liar!"

My adult son and daughter drove six hours to say those unforgiving words to me on August 1, 2013—a date I can never forget. I had envisioned our reunion as filled with hugs and kisses, after feeling a glimmer of hope as I entered the waiting room of my long-term rehab. Instead, my children greeted me with distrust, anger, and disappointment, refusing even to get out of their chairs.

During my rehab I had written them letters, though I never got any letters back. I felt this overdue meeting would re-establish a connection between us. But instead, there was only their hurt, the raw pain and disappointment on their faces as I listened to their words of fury for forty-five minutes. This was particularly hard because we had once been very, very close.

DEEP ROOTS, WIDE INFLUENCE

I am Danish bred and can trace my roots back many centuries. I like to think of myself as internationally based, with my siblings born in South Africa, Denmark, and Mexico, and my family settling in Holland, Denmark, Mexico, and the United States of America.

I was brought up in affluent Greenwich, Connecticut. There I was, captain of the high school swim team, a sport I continued at the University of Pennsylvania. My Filipino Malaysian-born father was an avid tennis player, so I followed in his footsteps, playing squash and soccer, attending twice daily swimming practice. I also held jobs as a lifeguard and swim coach.

Dad was an executive in the liquor industry, so in our house, alcoholic beverages were everywhere. It was the late 1960s and early 1970s, a world reminiscent of *Mad Men*. My parents partied, with their international, American, and Northern European friends, imbibing in excess, so it was accepted that my siblings and I would indulge in alcohol. And I did not disappoint. Although, I did obey the no alcohol code of rules for six months during the swim season.

After college, my stress increased. I got married at twenty-two and began my corporate career as a marketing strategist with Pepsi. I moved seven times for my job—Houston, Texas, the Carolinas, Florida, Connecticut, New Hampshire, and Virginia. I lived the life of a corporate relocation gypsy, a mobile life of pick-up-and-go, visiting my family on weekends, the only time I sobered up.

I would be productive until boredom set in. While drinking. I always felt in control, able to start and stop whenever I wanted. I could curtail my consumption for six months to a year. But when traveling, I was what you would call a high-functioning alcoholic, drinking only from 7 A.M. to 10 P.M., set and sober for the next day at work.

A SIGN FROM A HIGHER POWER?

I mentioned I had siblings, two older sisters, Suzanne and Maryann, and two brothers, one of whom was Thomas, an addict and alcoholic. For twenty-five years, Tom was in and out of rehab. He married three or four times and wound up in jail for forging prescriptions for pain medication.

When Tom died without warning of a heart attack related to his addictions, he was penniless, totally without family support, as he had irreparably damaged all relationships. This was a sign from a higher power, I thought, a warning, since he died on the same day, I entered my first twenty-eight-day rehab program. Like Tom, I couldn't get my act together. After his death, I often thought *if I had only known my brother better, I might have understood his struggle and hardships. We may have even supported each other's sobriety.*

DESPITE A YEAR OF SOBRIETY, I STARTED BINGE DRINKING ONCE AGAIN.

I quit cold turkey for over four years after getting a DUI in North Carolina, when I had to do community service and attend AA meetings, which made that stint of sobriety possible.

Then one evening I had a single glass of wine. Then two glasses, a few weeks later. Then three, and then vodka; I was a daily drinker in no time. I was not what you would call an ugly drunk; I was most comfortable drinking in isolation. I am a private person. Things weren't working well at home, no surprise. My wife didn't like my excessive drinking, and the children (now teenagers) were aware I was hiding bottles from them.

That pattern reminded me of my athletic career, where enough was never enough for me either. I was never good enough. I was never grateful. I was always searching for the next job, career, and athletic role, promising myself to be and do better next time. I was delusional.

My life was very scheduled. It had always been that way. At work, I was scheduling fifteen-minute increments to get things accomplished, writing objective lists, and even monitoring the length of time between bathroom breaks. When and where the next drink would come from was also carefully planned.

As a child and teen, I got kudos for all I was doing, as I was strong academically and athletically. And when my brother got in trouble with the police for drug abuse, the spotlight was on him. So, no one was paying attention to me.

CONTROLLING EVEN A FAMILY TRAGEDY

In the early 2000s, I got squirrely and decided to join a startup company. I commuted for a full year, all the while drinking when away from home. To the world at large, I didn't have a problem. Even the exciting challenges at work didn't reduce my cyclical inebriations this time, however. No one was paying attention, or so I thought.

Then, my brother-in-law died on 9/11 in one of the Twin Towers. No DNA was ever recovered. During those confusing and harrowing days, my family traveled to his hometown, Darien, Connecticut, to help keep things together. I appeared to control things while there, despite the reality that I could control nothing.

Soon after leaving Darien, I was back on the road with a new opportunity to do consulting for a firm in Buffalo, New York, with a good number of consultants reporting to me. My wife and I were empty nesters; our son was in college and daughter in boarding school. Since I saw how drinking influenced my performance at work, I stopped drinking for one year and decided on a new career focus.

Not long after joining the consulting firm, a CEO I had worked for previously recruited me to turn around a regional retail chain that had been acquired by a private equity group. But the challenge of turning it around was met relatively quickly and I recognized I was not growing, so I went in another direction—self-medication to relieve my perceived boredom.

Then in 2007, my wife and daughter went to Europe for a vacation. I picked them up at the airport, trashed, and they kicked me out of the house. I went on a two-day bender in a motel.

THE "SPIN-DRY" DETOX

As my bender continued, I showed up at work—again drunk. Disgusted, my CEO closed my office door, and the next thing I knew, I was being driven by the Head of Security and the SVP of Human Resources to a detox center where I stayed two or three days. Later I would drive drunk to a detox center in Dallas where they had a twenty-eight-day inpatient twelve-step program.

However, I realized very quickly that it was what they call a spin dry detox, that the platform would not address my psychological or personal issues. I needed to understand how this disease manifested itself in my life. I went through the motions but didn't engage in the program. With no sponsor to guide me, I thought I could still be in control enough to stay sober for a full year. White-knuckle sobriety is the name for when you're dry but not in recovery, and that was me.

One year after leaving the twenty-eight-day program, my father passed away. That certainly gave me that day's excuse to drink heavily. The compulsion quickly took hold of me, and I began hiding empty liquor bottles. During a Christmas ski holiday with my wife and kids, my son started marking the alcohol bottles, even as I continued drinking out of them. When I finally confessed after several hours of heated denial, I was kicked out of the house for the final time.

I moved to my sister's home, and the drinking continued. My marriage became a divorce. I tried detoxing for four days, but all hope and purpose for living had dwindled. Somehow, however, even without an AA program, and despite the immediate threat of relapse, I managed not to have a drink for the next two years.

ANOTHER LEVEL OF LOSS

Then, after two years, out of the blue, the drinking pattern started again. I moved to Virginia, where my mother had an empty home forty-five minutes away from where she lived. It needed work, so I brought all my belongings there and began working on repairs. But I continued to drink.

One Sunday afternoon, our caretaker ran to find me. The house had caught fire. Everything was destroyed. I drank all day long, knowing that I had lost my home, my possessions, my family, and me. I realized in my drunken state that I needed a rehab program lasting more than twenty-eight days, or I was going to die. I did extensive research and found a facility with an ongoing program; my plan was to stay six to eight weeks. I could get control of my life by then—that's all I needed. I had not stopped trying to control.

I took a train to this rehab center. It was May 18, 2013. I was met with some shocking revelations: I had to surrender completely to the staff's care and the facility's rules. No computer, phone, tobacco, caffeine, or candy. I was allowed one hour of television daily. I was strip-searched and evaluated medically and psychologically.

As much as I was still in denial, I was becoming a different person despite myself. Physically, I felt better, but mentally, I was still trying to control the length of time I was going to stay. This facility never told you when you were going to leave. But I had an end date in mind; I was staying six to eight weeks and that was that!

LETTERS I DID NOT WANT TO HEAR

Part of my therapy involved being in a group of four to six residents sharing challenges and progress. On June 20, I was asked to be seated as letters from my mom and siblings were read. The words were very stark, cold, cutting. I thought I had snowed my family, but the reality was that I hurt a lot of people. This was an eye opener. I couldn't hide, after all. People were looking.

The counselors had asked my children to write to me as well, but they refused, wanting nothing to do with me. That was devastating. I started journaling after hearing what my family wrote and discovered how much I had changed. But as much as I thought I was ready to leave, I was not given the okay. I had much more to learn about myself.

On August 1, 2013, the unexpected intervention I described at the beginning of this story changed my life. In a conference room at the rehab, my children vented their anger, disappointment, and distrust for forty-five minutes, telling me I had wrecked their lives.

After that meeting, I realized I could either walk out of the facility's gate and disappear or surrender to the program—to a higher power. I was never religious or spiritual, but I felt I was beginning to change.

I began to participate in coherent breathing, meditating twice a week in a group at the facility and on my own. I joined a yoga class that met twice a week, which helped me connect to myself on a different level. I also realized during these sessions that I had grown to believe in a higher power. Studying Eastern principles reinforced what I was doing and learning.

I got into running for an hour and fifteen minutes daily, and gradually I became intense about exercise. I look back now and think I had just moved from one addiction to another.

DON'T CALL THIS "EXERCISE"

My counselors held a big meeting about the intensity of my exercise regime. I sweat a lot when I run, so I got the nickname "Paul Puddles." But it wasn't trivial; my over-exercising was disconcerting to the staff because my behavior was unhealthy, addictive.

So, Paul Puddles was not permitted to exercise for one week. Being divested of this privilege, this rediscovered love of an exercise-induced adrenaline high, was too much to bear. So, I started exercising in my room, then running up and down stairs. But once it was reported that I was violating my enforced ban by using the stairs, that pleasure was also taken away—no stairs, no exercise. I was worried that I would re-gain the twenty-five pounds I had lost. I was even recording my weight-loss program and the distance I ran each day—a familiar obsessive-compulsive act.

I was told I could not do any exercise for two months. I was pissed. But I did what I was told. You are never quite there, even when you think you are. But I was halfway there. After 360 days as an in-patient, my counselors assigned me to a halfway house in DC—a real blessing, giving me time to look within and tour the sights too.

I worked out intensely but sanely. I started spin class twice a week, strength and core exercise on the TRX once a week and running when I could. And I attended more meetings around addiction, did service and community work, and even began dating. Life was more normal. I kept my weight off and did not drink.

I also began to understand how obsessive I had been; I was now finding balance. I began seeing little coincidences and receiving messages that made me feel really connected to something greater than me. Finding a penny on the ground meant something to me or meeting someone by "accident" that was really not an accident or hoping there would be a parking spot and lo and behold, it was there!

I learned a lot from my recovery. I discovered I have character defects; yep, I do. I didn't want to admit they were there. But I started being honest with myself, accepting myself where I was, right at that moment, being present, finding balance, and realigning life's priorities. I went back to the person I really am—open, honest, thoughtful, considerate, and childlike, mindful, and grateful for things. I can feel satisfied with what I have now. I don't have to run or hide or isolate myself from others.

I now believe things happen for a reason. I see how my addiction to alcohol can be easily replaced by other compulsions. So, I am more conscious about things now. I am consistently attending meetings. I go to an all-men's group where we talk about what's bothering us. We address spiritual issues. We have a supportive fellowship. We can relate. There is no hiding; we can see through each other's façade.

We can see that everybody's on the same journey. We're all recovering from something.

COMMENTARY BY MARILYN GANSEL, PsyD

FINDING BALANCE IN A COMPULSIVE WORLD

Compulsive Disorder presents itself as a repetitive unwanted pattern of thoughts, behaviors, and fears that interfere with everyday living. This disorder can cause significant distress prompted by anxiety. Alcohol abuse and its compulsion to continue this unhealthy behavior triggers more anxiety—often leading to depression.

Every day, people self-medicate with alcohol, drugs, and/or food. Their overuse of these substances provides temporary relief from the stress they are experiencing. Promising to stop these unfit behaviors is often futile, because the pause is not enough to warrant a cure. It takes a lifetime of self-reflection and support to recognize the triggers that causes a person to need "more."

Paul's journey to sobriety was arduous. His intervention and re-habitation program to detox clearly had its ups and downs. Temporary moments of success gave way, plummeting Paul into an alcoholic prison. There was no escape.

UNTIL . . .

Paul played sports as a kid. He loved swimming, squash, tennis, and soccer. But Paul never felt "enough" as an athlete. His low self-esteem and his home life, where he witnessed parties of adults drinking to excess, paved the way for his addictive behavior. When things got tough or when his job wasn't going his way, Paul thought he should drink to soothe and comfort him. Only, that treatment for his stress and anxiety wasn't enough.

So, in rehab, Paul discovered meditation and breathing techniques—tools to teach him relaxation. Then, he found exercise as the way to release his boredom and his endorphins. He uncovered a new way to get high; not intentionally, he substituted one addiction for another. The counselors recognized this; Paul was instructed to stop his compulsive exercise regimen.

WHAT PAUL LEARNED

Paul's obsessive nature, his addictive behavior, challenged him. Like the athlete, he over-trained, his "in the zone"—focus, energy, drive, and performance—making him feel unstoppable. He struggled to find balance in his life. Like most of us, juggling so many responsibilities and commitments, we run into overdrive. We then feel overwhelmed. Some of us do the all-or-nothing approach. Paul did it all when he exercised, not allowing his body to recover or relax. Paul may have been trying to avoid the real cause of his obsessive-compulsive behavior. But when he faced the *why*—the intrinsic why— of his behavior, he began to change. He recognized that he, like many of us, are recovering from something.

CHAPTER 6

GAEA'S STORY: MY HORSE, MY HEALER

"I very much go with the Buddha's quote, 'If death is certain, but the moment of death is not, therefore, earth seeker, what does one do with this very moment?'"

YESTERDAY WAS THE EIGHT-YEAR anniversary of my breast surgery. The following is the story of how I got to be here.

I found the problem because I had a mosquito bite under my breast. I was scratching the bite when I found the curious lump. I was with a friend who taught breast exams in free clinics, and she recommended that I get to a doctor quickly. I thought I would be okay. My father had died of a heart attack and there was no breast cancer in my family. Cancer was never on my bandwidth.

The diagnosis did come, however, and it was a humdinger of a shocker. I had a serious case—an undifferentiated cancer, and within a week, I had to have surgery. The lump was removed so that they could biopsy it to see what grade of tumor it was, how deadly it was, and whether it had spread.

The good news: it hadn't spread. The bad news: it was the deadliest kind. It was completely undifferentiated. Two of the oncologists gave me a 50 percent chance of living longer than two years.

I was never one to get lost in anxiety. But I had been, earlier in my life, a little vulnerable to depression. Working with mindfulness and meditation gave me a sense of bravery as I found my courage, expressed my love, and realized we all have limited time.

I deepened my Buddhist practice during my eight chemo sessions, spaced two weeks apart. I invited a friend from each religious tradition to accompany me to each session, to aid me in praying. I invited a rabbi, who is one of my dearest friends, then a Sufi, a Christian, a Buddhist, and an atheist poet. (I decided to cover all the bases.) The night before my surgery, somebody got news of it and invited 150 people from various communities, professional and artistic. They came to the Buddhist Center the night before to read poetry and sing songs.

They gave me tremendous support.

RETURNING TO THE WATER, THEN FINDING MY HORSE

As I was now neutropenic—lacking a certain type of white blood count—and unable to battle infection, I could not be out in public, so I had to give up my habit of swimming a half mile every day. After some time, and through meditation, I got back into my swim routine, so much so that, within one year, I took second place in a swim meet. This meant a great deal to me. It had been one year since my diagnosis.

Shortly after meeting a Tibetan Buddhist monk who worked very closely with the Dalai Lama, I developed a non-profit organization that I currently run. My first contact was with the Tibetan exile community. Knowing that life was short, that I really didn't know if I would live past two years, I wanted to use all the skills I have in service to humanitarian outreach. It was so very meaningful to me to integrate the mindfulness meditation, the neuroscience, and my thirty-five-year history as a trauma therapist in order to develop protocols in wounded communities.

I was still quite weak. I had no hair. I looked like a Buddhist nun. One day, a wonderful, retired lawyer friend from Los Angeles, Larry Silverton, in his eighties, my best friend's father, was listening to me talk. His wife had died of breast cancer, and he was inspired by my intention to develop this nonprofit organization. He was very wealthy and offered to donate to my venture. A Western rider, he said he wanted to go horseback riding with me, knowing I had fifteen years of riding and jumping experience. So, he rented some horses, and we went on a trail ride through the mountains as I filled him in on my plans for the non-profit.

THE HEALING POWER OF HORSES

I hadn't been riding for a long time, and I was a little weak, but there we were—me and Larry. He was eighty-three and I felt like I was seventy! When we got onto the flatland, though, Larry rode like he was twenty-five! He took off cantering like some ranch hand from the Wild West. I was blown away. He could ride the pants off me. I didn't have my chops. I was very tight, holding on for dear life. But I remembered how much I loved it. What a meditation it can be . . . what an amazing and powerful relationship with a being of such elegance.

I thought I might only have a little time left, so I wanted to ride every day. What if I applied my athleticism to this remarkable, powerful relationship with an animal and really developed the skills?

Screw the cancer. What if I met the goal by the time I was seventy? I could compete at the Grand Prix level! That was over five years ago.

As challenging as it is, and as scary as it can be, depending on the horse, there's a peace that you get from just being on a horse. There is a freedom in it. There's a remarkable sense of balance that you must achieve in your body, and an overcoming of fear that you have to manage in order to be a good rider. I would be at Training Level right now. Then there's First Level, Second Level, Third Level, Fourth Level, FEI level, Intermediate, Prix St. Georges, and Grand Prix. It's like going from kindergarten to twelfth grade.

I came back from LA and immediately signed myself up for lessons. I did love riding as much as I thought I did! I thought, *well, if I love it in a year as much as I do now, I'll lease a horse.* A year went by, and my skills progressed, and I leased a beautiful seventeen-hand thoroughbred, a grandson of Secretariat. I rode him for a year.

AMAZING SYNCHRONICITY AT STANFORD

Then I found out there was a Grand Prix Gold Medalist in my town, and I could train with her. The catch was that I had to own my own horse, so I bought a horse and I started to train. I worked for about two years with that horse before realizing that the horse wasn't suited for the task of dressage. I gave that horse away and invested in the most amazing horse, imported from Germany, the biggest purchase of my life outside of my house.

Her father was an Olympic dressage champion. I named her Tara, after the Tibetan Buddhist deity. Tara means compassion.

Through Tara, I learned to deepen my compassion. In whatever time I had left, I devoted myself to that. I now had two goals: to strengthen both my equestrian skills and my ability to be compassionate.

Oddly enough, at this same time, I was grandfathered into a compassion study at Stanford University's Department of Translational Neuroscience, where there is a medical center called The Center for Compassion and Altruism Research and Education. The Dalai Lama's principle English translator, Thupten Jinpa, created a secularized version of Tibetan Buddhist Monastic training, lasting nine weeks, that is being used at that center. It's being researched by neuroscientists and used in trauma trainings, stress reduction, and compassion building.

The Dalai Lama has partly funded this program, which also strengthens the immune response and helps prevent burnout. It felt more than coincidental that, as I named my horse Tara, I joined the first group of people to teach this protocol, which I'm going to do at the Department of Veterans Affairs for their PTSD units.

You must be completely present on a horse to be safe. Every breath you take—every step a horse makes—is new and different. You must be able to respond to that moment. This is a great teaching in strengthening our capacity to be extremely present. We also know from mindfulness research how important that is in terms of immunity and stress management. Elizabeth Blackburn did the research, winning the Nobel Prize in medicine a few years ago for her research on stress.

By working with impoverished, stressed mothers dealing with sick children, she determined that stress impacted the children at the genetic level.

Specifically, because stress reduces telomerase production, the telomeres, the end caps of the chromosomes, begin to fray. The end caps are what keep the chromosomes in place. When they begin to fray at the edges, you begin to see the diseases connected with longevity, like cancer, usually at ages seventy or eighty, but this happens at an even younger age to children who are underprivileged, when heavy stress played a role in their lives. Mindfulness meditation has been seen to have a good effect in such cases.

I moved into horseback riding eight years after my cancer diagnosis, well past the stressful marker of two years. I believe I'm here because I am doing these very strategic things that I love, that are deeply meaningful to me and give me great peace, but that also have some capacity to translate to the mind, body, and brain an overall sense of well-being. I think one of the keys in dealing with a life-threatening illness is that, on the one hand, you have to navigate and embrace your own mortality with some grace, humility, and intentionality. But on the other hand, you must also allow the challenge to be something that awakens you. You must live from an awakened place rather than a place that equates success with living or dying.

TO RIDE WELL, YOU MUST LET GO

I see my horse every day and ride it five times a week. Every day I experience an engagement with life that has been enhanced deeply by the lessons riding has taught me. If I want to ride well, I must let go. If you want to ride well, you can't hold on with your reins, or your legs, or your seat. You must let go and feel the attunement with your horse. If you want to ride, you cannot impede the movement of your horse. That means not getting in the way of your horse's essential athleticism, but instead, working with it.

Relax your thighs. Open your thighs. Cue with your calves. Differentiate essential body parts. At the same time, steer. Be aware of what you are doing and where you are going. And be aware of your environment. Is there thunder coming? Is there a storm brewing? The horse is going to feel it. He's going to want to run. He's going to want to pull you to safety. Relax! Don't be tense!

Horses can get scared. They are herd animals. If one gets really scared, that signals to all of them that there must be something to be concerned about. About six months ago, one of the horses got frightened. He must have seen a deer out of the corner of his eye. He just hauled off, galloping along a fence line to the place where I was on my horse, Tara's successor, a male. My horse then thought, *Oh, my God!* He has this very generous gentlemanly way of relating to me. He would never do anything to harm me. He would never buck me, or rear, or bite anything. He adores me, and he's my protector. He's my warhorse.

He was thinking, *I've got to get her to safety as fast as I can!* So, suddenly, he just takes off galloping. Now I'm riding a torpedo. He ran at a flat gallop for about half a mile. I was determined not to fall off. I just realized that all I had to do was calm him in order to calm the situation down. I took both reins in my hand and stroked him and said, "Easy boy, easy boy." He calmed down and came to a full stop.

MEDITATION SKILLS KEPT ME SEATED

My horse had a similar reaction later that week when we were riding in an arena and out of nowhere, thunder, a burst of lightning, and a downpour hit the metal roof. Being a German horse, he had never heard metal roofs sound like that. My riding skills were challenged again. A bronze medalist happened to be watching when these incidents occurred. The medalist was amazed. I told her that it's not my riding skills that kept me seated. It's my meditation skills. It is a very strong skill to be able to drop down to my center of gravity and stay calm in order to make my way through the moment. I think what happens with me when riding, and why it's been such a tremendous resource during this whole period of illness, is that I have learned to "worry well."

Cancer could return at any time. I'm not unaware of that. I may be closer to the norm now in terms of the risk factor for cancer returning. But the awareness is never something that goes away. Every six months, I have my blood drawn, and every six months, I celebrate the fact that there seems to be no indication of cancer in my body. If it were to return as a fatal metastasis, a brain metastasis, or as lung, liver, or pancreatic cancer, I very much go with the saying, "If death is certain, but the moment of death is not, therefore, earth seeker, what does one do with this very moment?"

HOW CAN I STRUCTURE THIS CHAPTER OF MY LIFE? HOW DO I LIVE EACH DAY?"

I choose to have a very noble beast, along with two great pups, in my life. I had named my mare Tara, meaning compassion, and I gave compassion away. This time I named my new horse Samadhi, a word that in Hindu, Buddhist, and Sufi traditions means the highest state of awareness. It's a kind of peace, bliss, and heightened consciousness that includes compassion, but goes beyond to a kind of deep wisdom.

Each day, as I engage with him, I see a little brass plate reading "Samadhi" that's tacked into his leather halter. His nickname is Sammy. Each day when I put his halter on and lunge him or ride him, I'm reminded of Samadhi and what it takes for us to be in our lives facing death with the intention of awakening.

SAMADHI MOURNS WITH ME . . .

My mother passed away one day in May. Earlier, when she was released from the hospital to go back to the nursing home, I flew out to Los Angeles, where our family gathered.

Before getting on the plane to go to LA to manage getting her into hospice, I went to ride that morning. I was so sad. In fact, I thought maybe I shouldn't ride because I was a little preoccupied. I hadn't slept all that well the night before, so I wasn't all there. I had my mind on getting on the flight. This is not the best state of mind for riding, when you really should have all your wits about you, especially with a horse as powerful as Samadhi.

As I headed down to the barn, he could hear me walking toward him. From a distance I could see him turning his whole big body around to look out the window, then putting his head over the stall and looking down the aisle to watch me come. He was eager to see me.

When I came to him, he licked me all over. He licked my face, my eyes where my tears were, my hands. He rubbed his cheek on my cheek. I said to him, "I am really sad today. You're going to have to take it easy with me." He continued to lick me. Then I realized how much I did want to ride, so I got my saddle, I tacked him up, and we went into the arena.

. . . AND SHOWS ME A SMOOTH TRANSITION

I had been working on making a smooth transition from the trot to the canter, and then from the canter back to the trot, to make it look seamless. My trainers and all the advanced riders say it's all about the leg position. Your legs need to be long enough to scoot under his belly and lift him into the canter if you can. That sounds nice, but I had never experienced it—like women who haven't had an orgasm, they've only heard about it.

A lot of equestrians have these elegant long legs that seem to go on forever, though I don't have long legs. They don't wrap under my horse's belly. But I got on him and I took a deep breath. We started working in the walk, and then in the trot, and then I asked him for the canter. Suddenly, I felt my legs drop down. It felt like they grew a foot until they wrapped under his belly, and he lifted off into the canter.

It was like flying. I've never experienced that. Wow. It had felt good before, but this is what they're talking about. This is what all the fuss was about. It was like, suddenly, I could lift him. He wanted to give me something different on this day.

He was tuned into me from the moment he felt I was coming and saw that he needed to lick my tears.

Samadhi and I had just lifted each other—body and soul.

COMMENTARY BY PAUL SCHIENBERG, PhD

GAEA'S RIDE WITH HER MORTALITY
FINDING CANCER

It was a decade ago that Gaea had breast surgery. There had never been breast cancer in her family. So, the diagnosis was a shocker. It was a serious case of cancer—undifferentiated—and within a week she had to have surgery. The good news was that it hadn't spread. The bad news was that it was the deadliest kind. Oncologists gave her a 50 percent chance of living longer than two weeks.

MINDFULNESS AND MEDITATION

Mindfulness and meditation practice gave her a sense of bravery as she found her courage to face her illness. Gaea realized that we all have a limited time on this earth. This awareness gave her a greater ability to express and receive love. She did not want to waste any opportunity to receive and give emotional support, especially in times of great need.

So, Gaea deepened her Buddhist practice during her eight chemo sessions which were two weeks apart. She invited a friend from each religious tradition to come with her to each chemo session. The night before her surgery, 150 people showed up from various communities, including professional and artistic. They went to the Buddhist Center the night before the surgery to read poetry and sing songs. They gave her tremendous support.

SWIMMING

Due to the chemotherapy, she had a lack of white blood cells that left it more difficult to fight off infections. She could not go out in public until the white cell count improved. She had to give up swimming. After a while, her white count improved. Meditation played a significant role in the improvement, and she was able to get back into her swimming routine and entered swimming meets. This was very important to her. It had been one year since her diagnosis.

PAYING IT FORWARD AGAIN AND AGAIN

Gaea wanted to give back support to those who were facing their own traumas. So, she came up with the idea of developing a non-profit with a Tibetan Buddhist Monk.

She did not know if she would live past the next two years. Regardless, Gaea wanted to use all the skills she had in service to a humanitarian outreach. It was so meaningful to her to integrate mindfulness meditation, neuroscience, and her three decades as a trauma therapist into helping wounded communities.

The father of Gaea's friend heard her talking about her wish to create the non-profit organization. He had lost his wife and had a good deal of money. He wanted to make a significant donation to advance her venture. They went horseback riding into and through the mountains. She had fifteen years of riding and jumping experience. They talked about her plans while they were on a long trail with the horses they had rented. Gaea re-experienced the powerful relationship between herself and the elegant horse she road. She decided to ride every day that she had left.

Gaea did love riding and she decided to buy her own horse. She had a great two years with that horse and decided she needed a different horse for the task of dressage. She got a horse from Germany that was built for dressage that was very expensive. Gaea named it Tara which means compassion.

Gaea learned that she must be completely present on a horse in order to be safe. Each breath each step can be different and new, and you must be completely present. This is as true with humans as it is with horses.

It is very important to do things that you love and find deeply meaningful. If you want to ride well, you must let go—just like in life. In riding, don't get in the way of the horse's natural athleticism. The horse teaches us how to get out of trouble and not get into it. The horse is drawn to do the things that it loves, that its built to do. We can learn so much from the horse—choose not to fight our instincts.

We must be, in our lives, facing death with the intention of awakening.

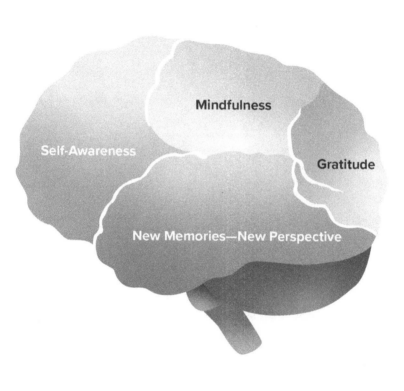

PART II
THE TENACITY OF AN ATHLETE

CHAPTER 7

JESSE'S STORY: JOLTED BY 13,900 VOLTS

"I chose to rise up, fighting with fitness as my way to recover, swimming many laps against currents of despair, depression, and pain."

IN AND OUT OF consciousness, I felt I was floating somewhere between earth and space. I was awake briefly, then asleep for longer periods, conscious for a few fleeting moments, then lifeless . . . neither here nor there. Losing consciousness would be truly a gift because what I was about to discover, after being in a medically induced coma for two months, would change my life forever.

Awakening slowly, I heard noises, but for the life of me, I could not place the sounds. Where was I? I struggled to move, to breathe, and to comprehend. When I finally put the pieces of what happened together over the next several weeks, I felt defeated. As I was gradually weaned off medication, I tackled mammoth withdrawal symptoms from the large doses of barbiturates pumped into my body. It was a living nightmare. But what I later learned after fully waking up was more terrifying, as I realized that my dreams of becoming a fashion and fitness model had been shattered.

FARM BOY TO FASHION MODEL

My farming parents raised seven children. I was the middle child who longed for a different life—one beyond the mundane existence I was destined to live. I had such big dreams. I guess I was quite unlike my siblings; I did not embrace the simplistic, religious, conservative life they accepted. I wanted more. Perhaps I was crazy or a bit uncontrollable. Whatever the label, I knew I had to chase my ambitions.

I left home at age sixteen against my parents' wishes. I moved in with a friend in Indiana and managed a construction company until I took the plunge and moved to New York City. Before relocating to the Big Apple, managing a construction company seemed a logical step, since I had acquired carpentry expertise from the farm and had been driving tractors since I was nine. Likewise, running a farm took business sense, so I gathered up my on-the-job abilities and strengths, applying them to this new occupation. But this wasn't my dream. This was not my future. My real aspiration? A modeling career.

It would have been easy for me to stay in Indiana, satisfied to be manager of a construction company. But I wanted more than anything to take the chance and live my dream. I wanted modeling to become a reality, and to do that, I had to give up the job I knew. If I didn't take the gamble and leave, I would always regret not trying.

So, at twenty-one years of age, I left my familiar world behind and embarked on a journey that, in only six short months, led to part-time jobs with Calvin Klein and Tommy Hilfiger. For me, modeling was easy. I just loved it. I had steadier work for a catering company between gigs, serving hors d'oeuvres to wealthy jetsetters. I was enjoying my life and looking forward to many years as a full-time, successful fitness and fashion model.

THE FERRIS WHEEL STOPS ABRUPTLY

But you can't always count on things going your way. Things happen; some things impact your life in such a way, you are not sure if you have the stamina to carry on. So my life, this fun, glorious ride I was experiencing, suddenly stopped mid-air like a Ferris wheel, swaying back and forth, hovering over the ground.

I learned you can't always trust people. I was a naïve soul, so on the night of December 2, 2006, after finishing a catering affair, I went out for drinks with people who I believed cared about my welfare—people I thought were my friends. I never thought that anyone, especially a friend, would cause me harm. It was going to be a night to celebrate, but instead of ending the night high on happiness and excitement for my next modeling job, it concluded with me running to catch the last train out of Penn Station, then lighting up the sky with my own burnt flesh.

As I ran toward the train, I felt different . . . weird . . . perhaps drugged (by whom, I didn't know), and then, as I tried to read the train station's monitor, my vision blurred. The next thing I knew, it was dark, and I was on the ground—or what I thought was the ground. My eyes focused on a metal platform in front of me. I turned sideways and saw the edge of a subway. I was lying face down on top of a stopped train. How did I get here?

Still woozy, I tried to steady myself. I needed something to hold onto—to grip—so I could get up and go home. My right hand reached up for a nearby rod. The minute I reached up, I felt a jolt of 13,800 volts rip through my body, cooking me, boiling me at 985 degrees! I lit up the darkened area, my shirt and backpack on fire. After a huge explosion, I heard my stomach roasting as the flames shot out from my face and shoulders. I screamed, and then choked on the smoke and fire. I tried to pull my fingers off the cable to release me from my living hell, and as I did, I fell eight feet onto the concrete platform. As I grabbed at my shirt and backpack, desperate to toss them from my body, my skin tore off with them. My right arm numb, I blacked out. I regained consciousness for a short time when I felt the spray from a fire extinguisher.

ALL I KNEW IS THAT SOMETHING TERRIBLE HAD HAPPENED

I thought I saw something in the distance. Was I seeing things? Were there people walking below me to get on the next train? I dropped onto the train tracks and stumbled across six of them toward the platform. Surely those people, if they were real, would help me. I tried to push myself up with my right hand, but it was useless. Then I realized why; it had fallen off my arm. I had no feeling at this moment. I only knew I must race against time, so I used my other arm to lift myself up.

Rising from the tracks, I screamed "Help me, please, help!" As soon as they saw me, the passersby screamed, too, and turned to flee. I could not imagine what I looked like to them, probably someone out of a horror movie. I didn't know it then, but my body had been melting away.

As sirens blared, I felt myself passing out but struggled to retain consciousness as a group of emergency volunteers appeared out of nowhere and placed me on a stretcher. As the ambulance wailed down the streets, I overheard the EMTs radio in, reporting that they didn't know if I was going to make it. Was I dying?

DEAD MAN, NOT YET WALKING

Apparently, I suffered burns over sixty percent of my body. The physicians at the hospital held little hope for my survival. I was put in a medically induced coma and given approximately two days to live. But miraculously (perhaps because I had been in good physical shape), my body fought to stay alive. Forty-eight hours later, a team of doctors began operating on what was left of me.

I AWOKE TO MY SISTER HOVERING OVER ME, WELCOMING ME BACK TO THE WORLD

I had been asleep for two months.

I wanted to speak to her, but couldn't, since I had undergone a tracheotomy and it caused an unbelievable stabbing sensation in my throat. I was also totally exhausted, even though I had been asleep for such a long time. Every little thing—every gesture, even blinking my eyes—was such an effort! I had lost fifty-seven pounds and had pneumonia from being in bed for so long.

I could not move my feet, hands, or neck; it took me several days to lift my head off the pillow. I was frustrated, angry beyond words. What was going on? Where was my right hand? I reached for my right arm and could not find it. Then, I realized the truth. My arm had been cut off . . . removed . . . amputated! I started to yell. Mom was at my bedside crying. She told me my arm was so burnt, it had to be removed. The doctors had no choice. I now had an elbow and nothing else. I would have been a dead man walking if I hadn't been flat on my back.

What was the purpose of all this suffering, this disfigurement? Why, God, and why now? I did not want to live. I argued with God! Why did you do this? What did I do to deserve this? Is it because I left home or wanted a different life? Was this a test of faith? Whatever it was, I didn't want it. My life was ruined. Nothing could restore who I was or what I had looked like.

Then the nurse removed my bandages, and I could see how ugly I had become. My skin was bumpy, my torso perforated. I was emotionally and physically consumed with incredible pain. I would later have to have multiple skin-grafting surgeries; it would take six years of stretching for my skin to mature.

I really felt I was being punished. I had to go to my family's home in order to be taken care of. I would never look like my old self.

I was a man without a future.

ONE FLASHBACK OFFERS PEACE, NOT TERROR

Like a Grade C horror movie, the accident began playing back in pieces. Memories of certain details began to haunt me. One of them was not scary, even though it came back vividly. It was a flashback that brought me peace. Seconds after reaching for the subway rod, I saw myself moving through a white tunnel. I also saw two doves and a large gate in front of me. I felt calm, peaceful, and loved. As I began to approach the gate, the white light dissolved and I felt pulled in the opposite direction, away from the doorway.

That's how close I came to death.

I was then brought back to a vision of my awakening on the platform, shirt and backpack on fire, my hand still clinging to the rod above me. I now know I died and came back in that instant. Why was I spared physical death when I felt dead—emotionally and physically? I don't know why, but God brought me back to earth. As I was approaching that peaceful light, I remembered wanting to go beyond the gate, but no, I was brought back to the hospital room, to my parents' home—an invalid bound to endure more suffering.

I later learned I died again at the hospital when my kidneys and pancreas shut down during my coma. The doctors revived me.

Why did they resuscitate me? I couldn't stand, sit, talk, or walk. I would have to learn how to do everything all over, like a child. Before the accident, I was right-handed; now I would have to learn to be a lefty. Because of my continual pain, medication was a constant requirement, to relieve the agony. I had no balance because of being confined to bed in a supine position for many months. Financially, I felt destroyed. Medical bills piled up. How could I earn a living and pay these bills? Originally, I was a strapping six-foot-two athlete in the best physical condition of my life, and now I merely existed as a bony, 143-pound, weakened person re-learning how to walk and write.

I prayed for death. One day, I tried not breathing. My face turned blue as I remembered the peace I felt in the white tunnel. But a nurse discovered what I was up to and stabbed my toe with a needle so the air in my lungs was forced to expel. I was back again in my hospital room—alive, not wanting to be there—wanting to close my eyes forever.

A NEW ARM AND A NEW OUTLOOK ON LIFE

And I also didn't want to move back home and rely on my parents to take care of me. Maybe, I thought, this is the way God was punishing me. "You're going home, Jesse, where you belong." But was He reprimanding me? I somehow felt I failed—that in some way I was responsible for my condition. I felt great shame, too. After all, I left home to pursue a dream I believed could be achieved. Now that dream was dead, like me.

My parents knew the depth of despair and depression I was facing; they were concerned I would harm myself, so they never left me alone. I felt judged by God, family, and friends. I was sinking; would I ever "swim" again? Could I ever be the winner I once felt I was called to be?

I started soul searching. Questioning God, my life, and dreams brought me to the awareness that I was not done yet. Somehow there was a purpose for this accident . . . for where I was right now.

Before the accident, I had been an athlete. I treated my body with great respect. After all, I was strong enough to endure 13,800 volts; my healthy physique defied the odds. Now I would have to decide to rise up or sink. Would I have the courage and fortitude to swim and fight for a new life purpose? Like fish swimming upstream, I would have to be determined, take risks, and adapt to change.

I chose to rise, fighting with fitness as my way to recover, swimming many laps against currents of despair, depression, and pain.

Once I wanted to be a fitness model more than anything, so I spent hours in the gym working out before the accident. Fitness was my sanity. It helped me stay focused and it raised my self-esteem. Now I needed more than ever to get back in shape. I realized I was not only handicapped physically, but mentally too. I needed to work on my mindset, my self-image, and discover who I was really meant to be.

When I was in the hospital, my mom promised that someday I would get the best prosthetic arm possible. Besides renewing the dream of becoming a fitness model, I envisioned my new arm. And while I did that "law of attraction" thing, I went back to working out. It was more difficult now because I was limited to lower body exercises and one-armed routines. But I did what I could—squatting a lot.

Then, after three years, I was fitted with a custom-made bionic arm from Hanger Clinic. It was the best arm ever! It gave me the ability to do pushups, hold dumbbells, and bench press. I found myself carrying groceries and driving a car and doing all the things I did before I had the accident.

I worked out for the next three years to improve my physique so I could feel and look like the athlete I used to be. I even competed in bodybuilding and fitness competitions. I participated in the United Powerlifting Association's lifting event, where I squatted 610 pounds using my prosthetic arm!

Seven years ago, I thought I had lost everything: my looks, my career, my self-esteem . . . even my desire to live. But, as I reflect on the agony and the pain and see what I have achieved with my new prosthetic arm, my new outlook on life, and my continued commitment to fitness, I see that I am here for a reason. I am here to be an inspiration to others, to mentor them on their path to good health. I am here to offer hope—to deliver the message that, despite suffering the worst tragedy that could happen, a person can overcome and realize all he's meant to be.

Today, I am a fitness trainer in Los Angeles. I still love to compete in bodybuilding contests and make public appearances as an official spokesperson for Manning UP USA—an organization designed to support survivors as they network and discuss how fitness can help overcome obstacles. I want people to feel empowered and stronger through sports and fitness, just as I did.

I also hope one day to develop a more innovative prosthesis for other survivors, so they may have more mobility to support their goals and careers.

I am Jesse, proud of rising, proud to help anyone fighting for his or her life.

COMMENTARY BY MARILYN GANSEL, PsyD

JESSE'S STORY TOUCHED ME deeply. Here was a young man whose dreams were shattered instantly by a horrific accident. His loss of limb and disfigurement from the electrocution left him in despair, depression, and pain. It is easy to understand why he did not want to live.

But what really moved me about his journey was his inner strength or power to withstand the pain and disfigurement and accept his loss with a new attitude.

Many of us have lost friends and family; but losing a piece of you—a limb—is a tremendous fatality. It is devastating from a physical perspective but also from an emotional mindset. His missing limb and burnt flesh affected his sense of identity and impacted his career as a fitness model— the aspiration he had in his early twenties. While he grieved his missing limb, coping with his grotesque physique and new thoughts of dying, his losses shifted into what he might take from this experience. He had the insight and resilient personality to continue pursuing his dream with a prosthetic arm and a burnt body. Jesse understood he had a purpose for living and enduring this nightmare.

He gave us an understanding of how a person can recover, rebuild, and restart his life and career—live a purposeful and resourceful life. Jesse gave himself attainable goals. He kept creating and finding new challenges as he brought his body back to life with exercise. He chose new habits; courage and fortitude were his fuel to adapt to change, take risks, and find a life of purpose. He showed us the importance of overcoming a detrimental psychological loss by pursuing self-healing activities. He drew on what he knew and loved to do—exercise and other healthy lifestyle habits to find positive meaning as he grew both physically and mentally stronger. He exhibited the truest form of resiliency.

Jesse's self-efficacy came from his strong belief that no matter what happened to him, he could still "bounce back" and be successful. He didn't have to have an education, certain income, or profession to exhibit positive change. His self-efficacy came from his commitment to exercise.

"The capacity for an individual to exhibit resilience may be determined by various influences such as education, income, and occupational status; however, according to Ryff[5] et al., (1998), the reflection of resilience is evident in the ultimate outcome of mind-body integration regardless of sociodemographic variables. Mind-body integration in this respect involves concern with positive mental strategies such as not becoming depressed, anxious, or physically ill in the face of adversity, as well as positive physical strategies such as diet, exercise, sleep, and aerobic capacities" (Psychophysiological Implications of Amputation, James Price, PhD, CPO, FAAOP).

Jesse is a role model, not just a fitness model. He is a superb example of finding purpose and meaning, gaining a new perspective, and choosing a positive outlook because of his disabling accident.

---

5   Carol D. Ryff and Burton Singer, The Contours of Positive Human Health. January 1998, Psychological Inquiry 9(1)

CHAPTER 8

EDMUND'S STORY: A DISABILITY DISAPPEARS ON THE SOCCER FIELD

I WAS BORN IN Ghana. According to my mother, I began walking at eight months of age, like many other children. When I was two years old, I had a life-altering accident. My female cousin was supposed to take care of me in her backyard while my mother left home for the village market. While my cousin was trying to cross a very huge drainage system gutter with me, a cloth of some kind that was connecting me to her got loose. I fell straight into the gutter and my cousin fell on top of me. That is how my problems started.

My parents tried very hard to make me better, but my condition kept getting worse and worse. This was in the early 1980s. They were giving polio vaccinations, but they weren't very effective. I was sent to a doctor at the Salvation Army missions in Ghana, and it was there that they diagnosed me as having the polio that started after the accident.

I underwent a surgical procedure because the doctor said the bones in my right leg were locked up. After the surgery, my parents were advised to take me for some orthopedic training and I was admitted to a hospital where I spent nearly five years, my mother taking care of me. I was taught how to use braces and crutches.

During the training, I spent several months on a bed with my legs hung up with some strings a good part of the time. They said this was supposed to help my legs straighten out. After that, I was given orthopedic shoes designed for people like me with mobility problems. I was also given a brace for my right leg, and it took a while before I mastered it. Soon I started to get around with the help of two crutches, the armpit kind.

I was discharged to go home with my mother and continued to go to the Salvation Army clinic nearby every Thursday. They provided transportation via Land Rover that would visit the small towns to pick up the children with polio who had undergone the same surgery. The other days, I went to school.

A while later, I was told to wear orthopedic shoes on both legs, even though only one leg was affected by polio, because the left leg had shrunk.

THE CHALLENGING JOURNEY TO "NORMALCY"

As I was growing up, I began to make certain decisions for myself. One decision was to stop using orthopedic shoes completely. I wanted to mainstream myself to join my peers. It was very difficult, because my mother wanted to follow whatever the doctors recommended. My dad took my side and wanted me to follow my own beliefs. Ultimately, they got me a pair of regular everyday shoes. The next step was to tell my parents that I didn't want the crutches. They tore the armpits of my shirts. I asked to use the elbow crutches—the ones that I am still using.

I was doing great in school, first junior high school and then senior high. Initially, my parents wanted me to be in a school that was primarily for people with mobility problems. I said no to them because I wanted to feel the way everybody feels at that age. I wanted to feel normal. I started at the school my parents wanted me to attend, but I lasted only a few weeks. I didn't fit in. So, I told my parents I wanted to change schools. Again, my dad talked to my mother, and they started looking elsewhere till they found a Catholic boys' school.

It was my first time being in a boarding school, and at first, it was very difficult trying to make myself known. I had to lobby for myself. I had to advocate to get somebody to give me some sort of help. For example, whenever the tap was not flowing, I had to ask one of my roommates to fetch a bucket of water from a pipe somewhere and bring it into the bathroom for me. It was an opportunity for me to become independent.

I started growing, growing, and growing. It happened exactly the way I wanted it, but I was still always on the sidelines seeing my friends, my classmates playing soccer whenever they had time after class hours. I had not completely accepted my disability. I kept asking God, "Why me? Why did all my friends have legs the way they wanted them to be?" They were running, doing whatever they wanted to do. I was the only person with mobility disability in that school.

Day after endless day of sadness, looking at them playing without me, I finally realized I had to accept my disability. It hit me that this was the only solution. It might not be the permanent solution to my problem, but it might uplift me and help me do things. So, one afternoon, I found myself accepting my disability. The next day, I approached my friends in that frame of mind.

"I'd like to play with you guys."

They said, "No."

SAME GAME, NEW RULES ON AND OFF THE FIELD

They were trying to tell me that there was no way I could play soccer because of my mobility issues, but somehow, during this back-and-forth conversation, they agreed to let me play. Then something dawned on me.

"When the ball hits your hand, it's a foul, right?"

"Yes," they agreed.

"How about, if the ball touches my leg, it's a foul, because I will be playing with my hands."

Initially they didn't like the idea. But one of the guys piped up and said, "I think it's a good idea. Let's give it a try and give him a chance to play with us. We'll see how it goes." The others jumped on board. So that afternoon as we all started to play, I put down my crutches and was crawling with my hands on the floor. As I "kicked" the ball with my hands, something wonderful happened. I was scoring more goals than all of them! I was able to do the corner kick and hit the post and sometimes the ball hit the top right corner of the goal where the goalkeeper could not reach it. From that day, they accepted me as one of the soccer players on campus—not with the soccer team but playing in a more leisurely way. They even wanted me to participate in their training sessions.

I WAS NOW A REAL PART OF MY SCHOOL COMMUNITY

That's how it started. From that point on, I was very involved in whatever they wanted to do and wherever they wanted to go. That made me forget my disability.

At one point, I asked the school authorities to bring my classes downstairs because I could not take the stairs, but they wouldn't move the class. So, I crawled up the stairs and made it part of my exercise routine every day. Eventually I graduated from that high school.

However, I could not go on with my education because I had no money. In Africa, most of the countries have a cash and carry educational system. You pay before you sit in class. So, I had to teach for a while, though the recruiters didn't want me to teach because of my disability.

I said, "Give me a chance." And they did, so I taught English and integrated science to junior high school students as a non-professional teacher. If you have a very good GPA, the government gives you the chance to teach elementary and high school. I taught for two years and accumulated enough funds to get into a tertiary school. I finally got admitted to the Ghana Institute of Journalism. However, after three people interviewed me, they noted that there was no way I could fit there, citing infrastructure barriers, insisting that the buildings were not accessible for people with mobility problems.

But "Give me a challenge like this and I'll be there" had become my motto. So, two years later, I graduated from the Ghana Institute of Journalism.

PICKING UP TROPHIES FAR FROM HOME

Ghana has a requirement that after you graduate from college you have to enlist in the National Service Secretariat with the Ghana Education Service. They give you a place to work, perhaps a school where you can teach or an administrative office. It could be anything. I opted to work with the Ghana Society of the Physically Disabled, with offices in Accra.

While working there, I was elected National Public Relations Officer of the Ghana Society of the Physically Disabled Youth Wing and held that position for a year.

When the DANIDA (Danish International Development Agency) came to work with the youth wing, it gave us the opportunity to apply for scholarships. I applied and was one of the few people in Africa chosen to study intercultural project management in Denmark. When I returned to Ghana after some months, I got a job as a project manager at a disability related center for the employment of persons with disabilities.

I was playing basketball at the same time, positioned on the front line near the basket, except when there was a problem in the backcourt, and then I would go there. Sometimes the coach wanted us to move around, then go out, then come back, especially when we played tough teams.

Every six months or so we played a West African sub-regional competition. It started when Ghana hosted about seven other nations, including Nigeria, Benin, Togo, Senegal, and Ghana. After Ghana won, we traveled to Algeria for a similar competition in which we placed third. We were having great fun.

I was still playing soccer as well, using crutches for support. I must admit I didn't put as much effort into that team.

At that time, I was living on my own in Accra while my family was living in the central region of Ghana. I rented a place that wasn't accessible, typical of almost all apartments at that time. It was very difficult. For example, earlier, I lived in a place where each of us had an individual room with a shower all our own, so I would have to remove my brace and crawl into the shower. It was very challenging.

THE SEARCH FOR MY PERFECT AMERICAN SPORT

I relocated to the United States in 2010 by myself after winning the US Diversity Visa Lottery in 2009 with the stipulation that I'd relocate in six months or lose the visa. I wanted to work with people who had disabilities and continue playing sports. So, the first thing I did after arriving in the US was to look for a disability related sport.

My internet search found Achilles International, which offered me something new to try—a hand-cranked wheelchair. I started training with Achilles in April 2010. I had several terrible accidents, but I continued to learn. An Achilles trainer taught me what I had to do, whether I was going uphill, downhill, or on level ground. Working the gears was different for each situation.

So, one day I was doing the hand cranking on my own. When I got to the west side of New York's Central Park, headed downhill, it felt like I was flying on the wind. Suddenly, I saw a four-year-old child crossing the road by himself. I could not allow myself to hit the child, so I intentionally fell, suffering bruises all over my face. Only recently have those scars healed. When you are going downhill, you must expect the unexpected. I got better and better at expecting the unexpected while going downhill and never had an accident again. Today I get the opportunity to teach new hand-crankers who would like to join the team.

I started going to school at around that same time. In May 2014, I graduated with a BA in social work from Lehman College. I have applied to Baruch College for a master's in public affairs, with the goal of working in public policy related to disability. From there I want to go to law school and become a human rights lawyer. I want to spend the rest of my life advocating for good services, programs, and policies for people living with disabilities.

I want to do this work, not only in the United States, but also across the world, especially in my country, Ghana, where the situation is, unfortunately, still very bad for people with disabilities.

COMMENTARY BY PAUL SCHIENBERG PhD

IN THE FIRST SECTION of Edmund's story, he lays out a remarkable series of traumatic medical events and treatments that exploded into the beginning years of his life. Some of these terrible occurrences were accidental, some biological and some intentional. None were created to willfully cause harm to Edmund. Edmund never thought of them as a victim of life. Nonetheless, the accident, the polio, the surgeries, the treatments occupied so many of his formative years. Obviously, they formed the major forces and the content of his young life journey. Along with the details of these horrific attacks on his body, a psychological theme began to surface.

Despite the best of intentions by a cousin to take care of him while his mother went to work, his parents getting him services he needed, doctors who did the best they could to heal his fragile body, orthopedic trainers to teach him how to use equipment intended to help him be mobile and overcome his physical challenges, sometimes they created more problems than they solved. Certainly, there were some gains that young Edmund made, but far from enough to have an independent life. He somehow concluded that he needed to take control of his life if he was going to thrive.

His mother wanted to follow the directions of the many doctors that tried to improve Edmund's life circumstance. On the other hand, his father was willing to listen to what Edmund wanted. So, his first decision was to stop wearing orthopedic shoes and his second decision was not to use the crutches that tore up his armpits and begin using elbow crutches. Edmund began to trust himself and listen to his body.

His parents wanted him in a special school for children with mobility problems. Again, Edmund revolted. He wanted to feel like everyone else. So, he went to a Catholic boarding school for boys. He was on his own and had to advocate for things that he needed to take care of himself, and he did. He learned how to manipulate his environment to get what was necessary for his body. With each physical challenge, he figured out what his body needed to thrive at school.

Edmund was growing normally. He was on the sidelines while his new friends were playing soccer.

But, one day he came to an important psychological position of accepting his disability, not in a defeated sense. He became friends with his whole body. He came up with an amazing idea; if the ball touched his legs, it was a foul, and he could use his hands to move the soccer ball. He turned the rules of soccer on its head, and he began to play with his friends. He learned to change the sports world to adapt to his physical condition. He scored more goals than his "normal" friends. Edmund became one of them and a full member of the school community. As a member of the soccer team, Edmund thrived. Team sports gave him a sense of himself as being a legitimate part of the school, his community, country, and the world.

A few years later, Edmund had learned how to play wheelchair basketball. As a member of one of the basketball teams, he traveled to many countries in Africa. Later in life, he moved to the United States and started participating in another sport. He found Achilles International. This organization gave him a hand-cranked wheelchair, and he learned how to use the gears from one of the trainers. Today he helps others use the same device.

Sports helped him overcome and give others the ability to use the hand-crank wheelchair. Team sports have given him the opportunity to give back what he had been given by others. Edmund learned that we all need help, and we all need to find our place in the world. Sports can help us achieve all these things and more.

CHAPTER 9

ALFONSO'S STORY: A BROKEN HOME MENDED ON THE BASEBALL FIELD

"I asked myself what a great son would do. He would embrace and forgive. And I did. Sports taught me that."

SHE CAME RUNNING ACROSS the baseball field, wildly waving her arms, screaming loudly, and smiling widely. The coach's wife wrapped me in her arms in a tight embrace. I was seven or eight at the time—the smallest player on the baseball team—and I had just hit a home run to right field. She planted a big kiss on my cheek, telling me how proud she was.

She was thrilled for me—me! My parents should have been at the game; my mother should have smothered me with kisses, and my dad should have said, "Well done, son." But no, here was a stranger showing genuine, positive emotion toward me. The feeling was overwhelming. I was somebody special. That was one message I got; the other was that people cared what happened on a playing field, and they cared about me.

I was special and I was surprised. I certainly did not feel that way at home.

BREAKFAST, CHURCH, AND THEN DAD'S BOTTLE

My parents, older brother, and sister were born in Mexico; my parents immigrated to the states when my siblings were very young. My father was a successful cattle rancher, a pioneer of the Mexican middle class. Not formally educated, my dad was handsome, dashing, and hardworking, but he also drank heavily. I guess I can't blame him for his addiction; after all, his own mother was a bit twisted. She was an alcoholic and would invite him to drink with her when he was a young teenager. The message! The influence! What an environment.

Anyway, there was a terrible drought in Mexico one year and everything my father worked hard for was destroyed—his cattle ranch, livestock, and self-esteem. The only thing left for him was his liquor until his brother, a union worker and homeowner in Chicago, invited him to come to the states to recapture normalcy and family health in new surroundings.

That was 1955. I was born in Chicago in 1958 and lived in that area until 1969. I would say that up to the age of eleven I came from a broken home. Dad was drunken six-and-a-half days a week. A staunch Catholic, the only thing he would sober up for was church on Sunday. We had breakfast, went to church, and then Dad got drunk.

My brother and sister played sports. I could see their teams as cohesive groups led by responsible adults, kids pushing to be their best. I witnessed a certain respect for coaches from the team. I, too, wanted to play an important role, earn respect, and have that same esteem for adults. I wanted to trust.

For eleven years, wherever I resided, I competed on all-star baseball teams, participating with kids older than myself. I excelled at the sport; I was always the best. I learned to lean on teammates and listen to a coach's guidance. It felt good; I knew what to expect as I assumed the role of a star, a leader. I liked it. I felt special then, but not at home with Dad, or even in the classroom. And I loved feeling number one; it gave me a sense of comfort and security. I learned to trust some adults, good people with no psychological baggage dragging them down.

I found a world of normalcy outside of family on the playing field.

IT ALL COMES APART

When I was eleven, my home life unraveled when my parents decided that if we moved to Mexico, maybe Dad's alcoholic problems would lessen. So, the five of us packed up all our belongings and drove from Chicago to Mexico City. Over the course of six months in Mexico, Dad found work, lost his job, and left our family. I didn't see him again until I was eighteen, when he was living in Las Vegas as a cook.

Moving to Mexico was hard. For one thing, I didn't speak Spanish and the language barrier kept me back a grade. When I was twelve, Mom realized what this sudden upheaval of my life was doing to me and enrolled me in an international school. One of the first things I did was join a baseball league that played year-round—eleven out of twelve months. To get to practice, I had to take public transportation to the other side of the city at all hours—alone. I would tell Mom my practice schedule and that I'd be back later. I felt responsible to my team. My coaches would be looking for me. I think back to what I did at such a young age, and I astonish myself. I was resourceful and eager to make things happen.

I received a tuition discount at the international school, staying there from middle school to my senior year. I played baseball, football, and basketball—an all-star from a broken home. I never had friends over to the house, and my parents never came to any of my school games.

I identified myself as an athlete and traveled internationally. I was on a Mexican all-star team, getting on airplanes to play games at sixteen, seventeen, and eighteen years old. I gained status and purpose. I was serious about my skills as an athlete. As a student at an international school, I hung around ex-pat families who were well traveled, experiencing different cultures and languages. I saw how normal families supported their children. All of this was a godsend to me. My athletic success gave me an identity with parents at the school; they would congratulate me on the game and silently wonder where my family was.

DAD RESURFACES

At the end of my junior year in high school, Mom told me that Dad had resurfaced in Chicago. He was dying of cirrhosis of the liver. Mom wanted me to go with her to see him, and I refused. She went alone and told me later that the doctors at the hospital said they had treated alcoholics for forty years but had never seen liver damage this advanced. He had gained thirty pounds of water weight and his intestines were exploding. Mom called each day, filling me in on his condition. Then, suddenly, his liver started turning around; he later said he had had a religious experience in the hospital after promising to do better if his life were saved. This was perhaps the only personal story my dad ever told me. He lived eighteen years longer.

But now Mom decided to move back to Chicago to be with him. *What about me?* I questioned. *What is going to happen to me?* Mom had it all figured out; I would finish high school at the inner-city school in Chicago. But I didn't want to go there. I had a married sister in Southern California and thought I could finish my senior year at her local high school. I never said good-bye to any classmates in Mexico. I just said, "I'll see you in six months," but knew I was never coming back.

I think I've learned *never ever say never.* After a few months in California, my sister told me she was getting a divorce, so I couldn't stay there. Where to go now, I wondered? I took a bus back to Chicago, where my only option was to enroll in a decrepit, mean-looking inner-city school. My parents lived in a one-bedroom apartment where I was to sleep on the pullout sofa. I no longer knew my dad. It was not where I wanted to be. Thank God, an aunt and uncle who lived in the suburbs of Chicago invited me to stay with them and enroll in a high school within their district.

It was springtime and baseball was starting. I was a bit disoriented at the school at first but gained instant respect on the team. I was an equal, excelling at what I loved best. Everyone accepted and loved me. They depended on my athletic ability. I was needed. I started to recognize a formula here. The structure of baseball as an athletic event was a way for me to contribute something of value, to be of benefit, to be important.

I was angry at my mom for leaving me, in a sense, leaving me to explore how to complete my last year of high school. My dad's alcoholism had caused so much damage. Now his sobriety essentially ruined my last year of high school as well! I was mad at them both because they could never really witness the role I played outside my family as an athlete. That is why sports were so important to me; they were a constant in my life.

I KNEW WHO I WAS WHEN I WAS PLAYING

Sports were everything to me; they gave me self-confidence, respect, and the accountability I yearned for. But the biggest benefit of all was that athletics paid for half of my college tuition. The summer after my senior year in high school, I brought eight or nine college applications to my mom for signing. I was accepted to all. I chose one university because some of my other friends were going there. Once there, I made the baseball team and received a scholarship.

I then realized the cycle of reward that came with hard work, self-discipline, and team spirit. In a sense, I was getting paid to play baseball. Wow. I was now identified as a scholarship athlete.

I played baseball for four years at the university and did well academically. I had found a new home. I had a strong need for acknowledgement that somehow, I was worth something. I needed an identity, and athletics and academics gave it to me. So, I drove myself to succeed.

I was happy.

EMBRACE AND FORGIVE: SPORT'S BIG LESSON

I could have been an angry young man, seduced by the excuse that I came from a troubled home, relocated many times, and had very little parental support. But I had the wisdom to know that an important element of a success formula is forgiveness.

We make mistakes during sporting events. And in life, you make errors. What do you do with mistakes? I asked myself. What would an outstanding leader do if he erred? You learn to forgive the failures of your teammates to encourage them on. You must also learn to forget your own mistakes in the game; otherwise, you will never perform to your ability.

I remember striking out during a critical part of a game. From my coach and leader, I learned you use mental processes to evaluate what a great athlete or leader would do in a similar situation. So, I learned to create in my mind a formula for how a great leader would behave—what he would say and do, and I would emulate that.

Sometimes it's easy to say "I forgive you"; it can slip casually off the tongue. But when you say *I forgive you*, meaning it authentically, genuinely, and from the heart, it takes on a new meaning. I forgave my dad by understanding that everyone has flaws; we are not perfect. I asked myself what a great son would do. He would embrace and forgive. And I did. Sports taught me that, and I use it today in my personal and professional life.

LAUGHING AT BIG UGLY OPPONENTS

I realized as an adult that I didn't have to participate in sports to apply what I learned on the field to business situations, particularly ones that seemed intimidating. But my sports experience made everything easier. Physically, I was always on the small side, so to beat bigger and faster opponents, I needed to outsmart them. My athletic prowess taught me to be faster, craftier. Even my speech patterns were quick. I learned that mastering fundamentals was the first step toward performing at the high level, where creativity and instinct take over. But I was never going to intimidate anyone, or so I thought.

At work, I found that the power that came with my position at the office could be intimidating to others, yet I never self-identified in that way. I expected a higher level of performance from myself and began to be seen as a teammate with authority. When faced with big, bad, ugly opponents, I laughed at them. I learned a lot of good things because of bad experiences. I was faced with challenges as a kid and now even as an adult as I saw opposition to my ideas at work. But I also knew how to get along and encourage others, how to master and teach the fundamentals. You can't be fancy until you own the basics. Without core values, you can't win a game.

I attribute my success as a leader in business not to talking a good game but to practicing hard, being fully prepared and thoroughly informed, knowing the details. Risks then don't seem so risky. This style I brought to the workplace is the technique I learned from playing baseball, where I discovered how to lead, support, and collaborate.

From sports I also understood how to be present in the now; how each experience can be powerful and influential, that it's possible to not miss a moment. I realized how important being there for a child is, that time is temporary, so I vow to do the best I can in any situation, but especially as a parent. I gained my identity through my positive attitude, my academic excellence, and my athletic successes. From sports, I acquired the skill to not allow challenges to inhibit my freedom or my success.

My life circumstances could easily have programmed me, but I decided not to let it.

Ten years ago, I was diagnosed with lymphoma. I clearly recall the day I received the cancer news. As in a dream, I found myself asking my doctor about my life expectancy. That week, I decided to approach cancer as an opportunity to demonstrate what living a great life with great adversity looks like, to live with a great attitude in the face of this circumstance.

I was laughing at my big, ugly opponent again. I had developed a muscle strong enough to win back even my own health. How I behaved with my newfound diagnosis would depend on my attitude.

What I discovered from playing baseball and failing at two major league tryouts was that my life wasn't dependent on winning each time; it was more about what I gained from my sport—my mental health, my identity, my education, my respect for rules and protocol, my physical fitness, my ability to manage my health. All this is priceless.

In the end, I always see myself as an athlete. But now I wear a suit.

COMMENTARY BY MARILYN GANSEL, PsyD

IN 1993, I OPENED my first personal training studio in Stamford, Connecticut. It was an exciting time for me. My enthusiastic clients, male and female, embarked on their journeys to get toned, lean, and muscular. Many sought remedies to lose weight. Whatever their goal, we strove together to make their dreams a reality. In some cases, there were proven successes; others struggled greatly, with a few finding their goal impossible to reach. Approximately twelve years later, I opened my second personal training studio in Kent, CT. At this time, I appreciated the power of the mind, body, and spirit as integral components to achieving and reaching goals. What is it, I wondered, that helped athletes achieve their goals even when life throws them a curve ball? How do they bounce back from failure, mistakes, illness, and injury?

As a student of applied sports psychology, I began to connect the importance of mindset practice and other techniques athletes used to overcome obstacles and move forward. Could the skills that athletes practice off the field be applied to everyday life for the non-athlete? Is there a hidden inner athlete in all of us that needs conscious awareness and rehearsal?

In Alfonso's case, his low self-esteem, nurtured by his participation and success as an athlete, changed his view of himself. He found a place where he was respected and valued. He saw himself as an athlete.

Visualization and mental rehearsal are key skills taught to athletes. They learn to see a play completed by rehearsing their routines over and over in their mind. They absolutely need practice on the field. But without precise mental training, performance in any sport often leads to missed opportunities for a win. Alfonso knew this. He also knew teamwork and forgiveness as valuable lessons that he could carry throughout his life—not just on the field. At work, he saw himself as a good leader, and at home, a good son. He mentally prepared himself at work for failures and mistakes, learning that he could use these experiences as opportunities for growth. All the sports skills he studied became like second nature and easily translated to his work environment.

Even Alfonso's cancer diagnosis didn't deter him from facing his opponent head on. He laughed—seeking to use this illness as an opportunity! All that he learned and practiced at baseball gave him opportunities to lead, support, and collaborate at work or with any challenge in life. It's not easy to be an athlete. It takes courage, resiliency, dedication, hard work, and sacrifice. But the lessons learned, as Alfonso attested, leads to success in the world. Sports give us a chance to change and grow, to be successful, to learn to work with others in a supportive way, to forgive and move on . . . while wearing athletic apparel **or** a suit.

CHAPTER 10

MATT'S STORY:
BULLYING, BASKETBALL,
AND . . . BADMINTON??!!

"Don't listen if someone tells you you're not good enough!"
"No one can make you feel inferior without your consent."
—Eleanor Roosevelt[6]

LIFE WITHOUT MATT

What would life be like without me? Would I be missed? Would my friends actually care if I was gone? These are some questions I asked myself at age seventeen when I thought of ending my life—when I had thoughts of suicide.

I was born July 19, 1993, in Syracuse, New York. We were a family of four: dad, a hard-working man, mom, a stay-at-home mother, and Nick, my younger brother. We were a typical middle class family attending church on Easter and Christmas Eve; home was my haven.

Other than that space, my daily world was the same routine; wake up, then go to school which I hated because I knew I would be picked on because of my nose and how big it was. Or I'd get teased about how my

---

6   PrintHappyStudio https://www.etsy.com

hair looked. Every day, there was some event around me for which I'd get bullied. Every day was hell for me.

ANTSY AND ACTIVE

I was such an active kid—very athletic, but also antsy. I was so restless, on the go twenty-four seven. I had difficulty sleeping. I wondered why I didn't sleep much; after all, I was so hyper-active during the day. Why couldn't I collapse at night and fall asleep?

Maybe my restlessness could be attributed to apprehensiveness—a lack of self-confidence exhibited on the outside as fidgety. So, I stayed full of zip, not aware it might be a cover up for my insecurities. My family encouraged me to play sports—basketball, baseball, and soccer. So, I remained occupied with athletics and school.

I supposed I took after my father in some respects—imitated his great work ethic. He started his day at 6 A.M. and was always doing something. I was always doing something. He survived on three hours of sleep. I didn't sleep much at all; maybe I had attention deficit hyperactivity disorder—I don't know. It was never diagnosed. But I was also influenced by my dad in very positive ways; he showed immense caring for others, demonstrated compassion by putting the needs of others before himself.

MY FAVORITE THINGS

School was okay but not particularly my favorite place to be. Despite that, I never missed school, because my favorite things were basketball and baseball. I struggled with writing assignments; mom had to edit my work because I made so many grammatical errors. When composing an article or essay, I used run-ons. I just didn't care about correspondence of any type. Literature and the composing that went along with the subject matters were not interesting. Language arts bored me. What excited me was my favorite class—physical education, because there, I was the gym class hero. At that time, I aspired to be a professional NBA player. I had high expectations and believed I would achieve that goal.

PICKED ON

Even though I felt like a gym hero in the sports arena, it seemed I was always picked on—known as the class clown. I guess I did some bizarre things. In sixth grade, for example, I jumped out of a school window to get a pencil that was thrown out the windowpane. Boy, was I teased! And then in seventh grade during tech class, we were playing Silent Bomb where we would sit on desks and throw a ball to a person in the room. I threw the ball to a girl. She missed the catch; so, I thought I would retrieve it for her. But the ball had rolled out of the room and down the stairs. I attempted to rescue the ball but instead needed to be liberated as my head got stuck between the stairs. The whole class laughed at me.

But there were also times I was tormented without provocation. In eighth grade, I got kicked in the balls by a soccer player named William. It was not an accident. I got hit in the stomach too; one ball left me in such pain, I had to go to the hospital for a sonogram and missed two days of school.

It seemed as if everyone made fun of me. I'm Italian and the Spanish kids had a nickname for me; "*Nariz Grande*," the kids would squeal, meaning "Big Nose." I blamed myself as the reason I got picked on every day. I always had a problem of not sticking up for myself. I never had a backbone or the words to fight back, to razz the teasers or insult my classmates as they did me. My brother had the words; I had the brawn. I was an athlete; I couldn't fight back with words. Fortunately for me, basketball was my escape from the world of bullies. I would get on that court, and I could just tune everyone and everything out during the time I played. I wasn't made fun of, judged, tortured, or ridiculed when I played. Life on the basketball court was great!

UNSAFE AND UNBALANCED

By the end of my junior year in high school, I was diagnosed with severe depression. Our family physician prescribed Zoloft which is used to treat depression, obsessive-compulsive, panic, anxiety, and post-traumatic stress disorders. Even though I was still playing basketball and felt I could remove myself from the bullying on court, I felt unsafe at school, a great angst about being there. Apparently, I later learned that my parents suffered from depression, so perhaps this chemical imbalance was inherited or genetically produced. Anyway, I was put on 25 mg of Zoloft, then 50 mg, and finally the dosage that I am still on today—100 mg.

During this time, I stayed home sitting in my room—wanting to be alone. From time to time, I contemplated thoughts of suicide. I thought about ending my life. I didn't think anyone would care. My classmates told me they had my back, but they didn't. Friends who I thought would be there for me—stick up for me—just joined the bullying. My parents could see the dramatic change in my personality—my need to retreat—and they were devastated.

In my senior year, I finally saw a therapist. For the first time, I began to talk about my feeling and aspects of my life. I shared thoughts about my family, friends, and interests. I didn't reveal any reflections with my family or friends, because I didn't trust them. With my therapist, I could cry when I needed to. I guess I couldn't talk or cry with my family because my dad had a short fuse. He didn't talk much, and like me, he had little or no patience. Now that I think about it, I am the spitting image of my dad; although now, after therapy and the right medication, I am exhibiting more of my mom's qualities. I also believed if I shared my innermost feelings with my parents, it would be an extra burden for them. So, I kept things inside me—stored up, ready to burst open. I was a people pleaser, but no one pleased me; no one at school gave me a break, so I kept to myself, sharing what was really on my mind with my counselor.

FRESHMAN, FRESH START

I was accepted to Adelphi University. As a freshman, I was given a new start which really boosted my self-esteem. I had no old friends to bug me, no past to haunt me. I was away from the drama and fakeness of friends and high school. I was so excited to begin afresh! I decided to major in psychology with a minor in sports psychology. I thought I might become a counselor for middle school students—a way for me to give back, to make a difference. Adelphi had a well-recognized psychology program, and I was eager to learn. I also thought about becoming a gym teacher or personal trainer. I loved kids and believed I could help them. I didn't think much about becoming a professional sports person that year. My sights were set somewhere else now.

WHO WOULD HAVE THOUGHT—BADMINTON?

So, in my sophomore year at Adelphi, I found I was quite good at—of all things—badminton! Matter of fact, I was a strong contender. Now, mind you, I could play any sport, although I am not a fan of contact sports except basketball. Here I was on a badminton team in college and the president of the club told me, "I'm so glad you joined. We needed some good talent." What a needed boost to my ego; by senior year, I am the president of the badminton club! Who would have thought?

For once in my life, I felt appreciated by others—part of a team where I immediately was ranked the top third on the team!

I also began weight-lifting my freshman year of college. I was nervous about beginning the training at first. But a close friend encouraged me to go with him and I did. Not too long after, I began to get ripped! I got stronger physically—really got in good shape—but more importantly, the stronger I got physically, the stronger I became mentally. My newfound appearance boosted my self-confidence and weight training was a great stress reliever for me. I would rush straight to the gym after classes, Monday through Friday, where I would get such an adrenaline rush.

I majored in sports psychology. But, I found out in my senior year of college that I had health problems. I wanted to go to graduate school which put additional stress on me, while health issues got worse.

HIP DYSPLASIA DIAGNOSIS

It seemed that suddenly out of nowhere I started this hip-swaying movement when I walked. Any side-to-side movement hurt; the pain became so excruciating, it ached to sit.

According to the encyclopedia, "Hip dysplasia means that the hip joint is the wrong shape, or that the hip socket is not in the correct position to completely cover and support the femoral head. This causes increased force, and abnormal wear on the cartilage and labrum."

I started receiving shots to the area, but that didn't help. So, the osteopath chose to operate by going into the hip, cutting the muscle and tissue off the bone, and screw the hip back in place. Eventually, when I am fifty or sixty years old, I will need a hip replacement. The cause of this health problem could be genetic, or it could be environmentally caused by overexertion from sports, for example. I am not sure what caused this hip socket from dislocating, but I knew then, quite positively, that any thought of an athletic career would not be possible.

WHEN THE GOING GETS TOUGH

There is a saying "When the going gets tough, the tough get going." Well, I had a saying "When the going gets tough, give up." And I was ready to pack it in, just curl up and die, when I was in high school. I stayed in my room, until one day my parents confronted me—cornered me and made me talk about my feelings. And in doing that and talking about school issues, my eyes were opened. I thought about my family who loved me and the sports I truly prized. I started thinking, *I can't give up. I must fight for what I want. I have to become more focused.*

So now I was given a tough medical diagnosis, challenging surgery, and a difficult recovery, but I knew from studying sports psychology, I could do more than cope. I could lead a life of determination, helping athletes with their pre-game jitters and nervousness. My sports psychology tools and my own life experiences with bullying could prepare athletes mentally as well as physically. My newfound wisdom would teach them to stay in the zone and focus on the task at hand, turning off internal emotions and messages that say, "You can't. You always freeze in this situation." I could help them in controlling their emotions, their anger and frustration; I knew what it was like to play a sport, and what can happen if your temper or senses become overwhelming.

WHAT BULLYING AND SPORTS TAUGHT ME

Going through difficult times can teach you something about yourself—even bullying. After college and my operation, I learned, first and foremost, that I was ready for the real world. I learned little techniques from my therapist, my mom, and sports psychology—how to use coping mechanisms like badminton and mental rehearsal to overcome difficulties and teasing. I learned self-confidence through my basketball and badminton triumphs. I also found self-esteem by choosing friends more wisely, being selective about who I could trust. I learned I could surround myself with supportive people and parents.

I discovered that we can all have a fresh start in life. Those sports gave me confidence. My therapist, parents, and the newfound friendships gave me support and encouragement; now I can pass all that on to athletes and kids—especially those who feel bullied and want to end their life.

COMMENTARY BY MARILYN GANSEL, PsyD

WHAT TO DO WHEN YOU BELIEVE YOU'RE NOT ENOUGH

I was always the shortest girl in my class, both in elementary and high school. So, as a result, I was always selected to be in the front of the line, or in the front seat. I hated being singled out to lead the line. I wanted to experience the back of the line or the seat in the back of the room—at least once.

I was also the shyest student, probably because my learning disabilities made reading, comprehension, and retention so difficult. So, like Matt, feelings of inferiority and insecurity were my closest companions. They, along with some teachers who felt they could accurately predict my miserable future of failure, contributed to the persistent realization that I was not as bright as my classmates. I could never measure up.

It soon became clear to me that I was not going to be a math-wizard; forget geometry. Science, except for biology, was not a subject in which I excelled either. School was boring—and frightening and so restrictive—sitting at a desk all day, listening, writing, reading. Plus, I had to put up with negative thoughts about the story already written for me: "You are not enough. You will never go to college." It was like a death sentence I carried inside my head. I held myself as if I was invisible, head down and shoulders slumped. I chose to daydream. I wanted to be outside, ride my bike, climb trees, and be free. I was not the smartest person in the world (according to the schoolteachers), so how was I going to succeed in life?

My low self-esteem and low confidence dramatically impacted how I retreated into myself. Matt also felt safe in the security of his room away from ridicule and away from school. He suffered from several negative consequences as a result of bullying, including low self-esteem, depression, anxiety, suicidal ideations, and self-harm. Matt became self-critical, believing that he lacked the ability to cope with torment and rejection.

He had no coping mechanism. He walked like a loser, talked like a loser, and thought like a loser. His script was well-rehearsed.

COMPETITION IN SPORTS BUILT CONFIDENCE

There are ways to turn negative thoughts and messages into positive ones. As the new messages of confidence become ingrained in one's mind, another habit is formed instilling positive thinking skills. For Matt, badminton opened the door to believing in his abilities as an athlete.

He began to strut like an athlete, building his resiliency with new ways of thinking. He learned to change negative thoughts like "I really blew this game" to "I did my very best today. What have I learned that can adjust my performance next time?" He began to enjoy competition, and his inner athlete appeared ready to take on the next athletic challenge.

EXCEPT . . .

Matt never imagined hip dysplasia his next athletic feat. He could have fallen for the *poor me* syndrome. But competing in sports taught him core values that sustained even the worst health diagnosis. His sports psychology studies also proved essential to building more coping mechanisms. Just like an athlete who faces devastating loss or injury, he used mental rehearsal to see himself as enough. He began to turn his "loss" into opportunities for continued growth. He discovered new strengths and built his confidence with supportive friends and family.

EASY TO RELAPSE

Like any new habit, we become comfortable and return to old habits. Every athlete knows that thoughts become actions—that to stop those pessimistic thoughts, takes daily practice. Matt's determination and resilient mindset changed the way he thought about himself and his talents.

For me, I was going to choose to discover my strengths, nurture a positive self-image, and look at my problems rationally to find the best solution to solve them. I decided to maintain a hopeful outlook filled with gratitude, joy, and good self-care; working out several times a week saved me from self-doubt and depression. I developed greater resiliency because I, like Matt, chose to learn and grow from difficult situations.

I know today that I would not have been an exceptional elementary and high school teacher or entrepreneur had I not experienced the difficulties to learning. My creativity—my great strength—afforded me ways as a teacher to reach youngsters who also lacked the writing, speaking, and critical thinking skills as I did. Together, we designed new ways of learning that were fun, innovative, and exciting. How thankful I am to have had such an opportunity to struggle in school, and how thankful I am for my size as I can relate to those of us who need stepstools to open cabinets well out of our reach. Of course, I am most grateful to my trainer, Sally, who awakened the inner athlete in me.

I know from life experience that people who feel inferior—and who have not practiced coping skills—feel like losers. Struggling to be at the top of their game, they often persecute, bully, and mock. They attract and associate with those who feel the same pain, hating others and finding comfort in making others their scapegoats. They will use any means to mask their feelings of inferiority and elicit the illusion of superiority.

Too bad they haven't realized that no one can make you feeling inferior without your consent! You are already ENOUGH!

CHAPTER 11

JONATHAN'S STORY: THE ALCHEMY OF EXERCISE AND INNER POWER

"It came to me like a bolt of lightning—something possessed me this time. Today is going to be different."

I WAS VERY ISOLATED and shy as a teenager, struggling with a lot of social anxiety. I never felt like I belonged—something many kids go through. I was a well-intentioned person in grade school and wanted to be friends with everyone. But there were dark motivations and a deep-seated rebellious drive inside me. In part, this rebellious streak was born because of the way I was treated in the family. I loved my parents, and they did a good-enough job raising my three sisters and me. But, at the same time, I wasn't recognized for my skills or encouraged to use them. I was a high-energy boy in a family of mostly females. My father worked a lot of the time. So, I socialized like a girl. That was a problem, because, clearly, I wasn't a girl.

Many problems are created in Western culture by a "fundamental divide" that is placed between teacher and student. It all too often instigates a very authoritarian and rebellious dynamic, which has always rubbed me the wrong way. Most teachers tell us that we must do things "because I say so," offering no rationale for those assignments, rules, methods, and tests.

As a result, I hated school. The teachers were one-sided, one-dimensional, and thought they were great at what they did, but in reality, they were not. That, coupled with my normal teenage rebelliousness, planted the seeds for what germinated later in my life.

BRINGING MY MEDICINE TO THE WORLD

In high school, I stumbled onto the path of drug abuse through the hip-hop world, which was more of a religion than it was a subculture. I started smoking pot to self-medicate and calm down. It was hard for me to understand what was making me feel so anxious and uncomfortable back when it all started. I do remember one of my best friends saying, "You are a lot less angry when you smoke pot." That moment stood out in my mind for years. But I didn't know why I was so angry, and why I felt so out of place, like I didn't belong anywhere.

Drugs and hip-hop were my social lubricant. I got acquainted with graffiti art and free-styling and, more important, the people who became my friends. They also smoked pot—a lot of it. Pot led to other drugs, and that really spun out of control. I was making bad decisions and exhibiting self-destructive behavior. Here are just a few: drinking and driving, smoking pot and driving, using hallucinogens and driving—which I knew were completely insane. Then I got into a lot of fights and started dealing.

Believe it or not, I thought I was doing the right thing—rebelling and creating my own way of going about life, not just buying into the things that I had been "force fed" through the education system. In retrospect, I'm glad that I went through all of that because it taught me a tremendous amount about myself and about my resourcefulness. At the same time, I was very out of control and hurting myself and other people who cared about me the most.

A rite of passage is often in play when we test ourselves. In many ancestral and indigenous communities, an entire tribe will be there to support a male becoming a man as he tests himself. The elders guide the young man on the path of discovering who he really is and what value he could bring to the tribe. This is tradition and transpires during mid-teenage years—right around the time I started using drugs. I now refer to this part of my life as my "rite of passage."

Many contemporary high school children are facing these issues without mentors or elders to guide them, yet the elders and these rites of passage are fundamental to one's development. I grew to understand that, deep in my psyche, some part of me needed to die to create space for another part of me to be born. The problem was that I had not found elders to guide me.

So, I went on a very dark and self-destructive rite of passage and made it out alive. Not all my friends did. I'm glad I did and was able to use those experiences to bring my truth and my medicine to the world.

When I was seventeen, I really began to aspire to change. One day, as I looked in the mirror, I said to myself, "I don't know why I'm doing this, but it's me doing it, therefore I can stop." In that moment, I had created a daily ritual that would start my journey into a healthier life. It came to me like a bolt of lightning—something possessed me this time.

FITNESS HARNESSES MY INNER HIGHER POWER

Today is going to be different. I had said that so many times before, and then smoked some pot, took hallucinogens and opiates or ecstasy, or mixtures of several other drugs. I struggled with them for a long time. This time, in that moment in front of the mirror, in that awakening, that statement came from a deep unconscious place. It was me, but it was not me. It was both. It was something moving through me for sure.

It wasn't some outer higher power. I don't believe in that idea. I believe that the higher power is inside of us. That's what the moment in front of the mirror felt like. My inner higher power came out and allowed me to experience that profound moment. It wasn't joy, but it was clarity.

I decided to go away to college. I thought a change of environment was just what I needed to better influence my behavior. It was transformative to be in a new environment and to have this clear commitment to myself.

I didn't know what I was going to do with it or where I was heading, but I had that clear commitment to myself, and I didn't have all those old friends egging me on to old, destructive patterns.

There was this girl I fell in love with. She was only into guys who were fit, who worked out and had big muscles. So, in that freshman year of college, I didn't do any drugs. I just worked out with passion, commitment, and dedication. It transformed me, and not just physically. When I came home the next summer, I felt like a different person. I felt strong and confident and clear-headed and more valuable. I wasn't messed up, and I believed that I had something to offer others for the first time in my life. By the way, it didn't work out with the girl, but the experience was worth it. I discovered how to harness that inner power.

During that first year of clarity as a freshman, there was someone I met whom I thank to this day. He was a walk-on athlete for the football team at Villanova. He was a big, strong guy and started teaching me a lot about weightlifting. I have been weight training for thirteen years now. Over this period, I have had the opportunity to be trained by world-class coaches and thought leaders. They brought many good things into my life, leading me to make the best decision of my life. At age twenty, I decided to become a personal trainer.

PAIRING EXERCISE AND SPIRITUALITY

I didn't stay at that college. Instead, I came back to New York City to study at New York University in Manhattan. I was a sophomore, needed money, and wanted to have a gym membership. So, I walked into a gym near my classes and begged them for a job. That's how I got my start.

By combining exercise and spirituality in a unique and authentic style, I created a training program that is customized and designed for each client. My brand is called Train Deep Exercise Alchemy. It's about the deeper aspects of working out—how you can use exercise to become the best version of yourself in every aspect of your life. I designed the brand as a reflection of my life experience.

I finally found great elders who mentored and coached me along the way. For example, Tom Horowitz was a biomechanics and exercise mechanics expert in Oklahoma. I flew there four times to study with him. Another exercise specialist from California focused on holistic fitness and made a profound impact on my training program. I also learned from yoga teachers, and Tai Chi and Qi Gong instructors. A few of my teachers practiced Native American traditions. All these approaches have been integrated and are distilled into my brand and are very evident in the way I approach helping someone reach his/her goals. I teach myself as I learn how to teach others.

I have changed a lot through being a coach, a personal trainer, and a mentor for other people. That's the magic of it—it's a two-way street.

When trouble comes, as it inevitably does in life, it is an ordeal, a trial, and, as some indigenous tribes refers to it, "a dark night of the soul." This is when life really tests us. Victor Frankl, who survived the Holocaust, once said, "When we are no longer able to change a situation, we are challenged to change ourselves." I have changed so much in the way I approach struggle and suffering.

Now, I accept that life presents emotional and physical challenges to all of us. I have come to understand that I was meant to go through them to learn how I can use these situations to get what I want. Often, the most trying situations are where we really find out how strong we are. These are the situations where I find alchemy. It's taking the poison and turning it into medicine. There is a lot of magic in it. In looking at life from this perspective, I see challenges as invitations to become even stronger.

The second major challenge came when I got a herniated disk in my neck. I was twenty-six years old and thought I was on top of the world. I was strong, making money, and helping people. All of it was snatched away when my neck got injured. From the simple act of drying my head too roughly with a towel, I suddenly had the neck of a ninety-year-old. I was brought to my knees, but I owned the problem, just like I owned the problem of drug addiction. I gained strength from the fact that I had already been through an ordeal and had succeeded in turning it into a positive.

But this neck ordeal seemed harder for me; I was going to have to change careers.

It took me a good two years before I got on the right path for the solution. I went to doctors who recommended surgery. That approach didn't resonate with me. I decided on physical therapy, which resolved my neck pain and taught me a great deal about my body.

While on this journey, I developed an amazing relationship with a one-in-a-million physical therapist who not only treated me, but he now treats my family, clients, and friends.

SNOWBOARDING AWAKENS CHILDREN'S FEARLESSNESS

Mentoring is a large part of my life. I am very moved by kids who are struggling to find themselves. I volunteer with an organization called Stoke Mentoring. It is a nonprofit organization that creates the opportunity for children to safely experience their own power and realize possibilities.

I teach inner city kids how to snowboard. It wakes up something inside of them. They face their fears of getting hurt. They come to realize that our bodies have been designed to learn through movement and through play in natural environments over hundreds and thousands of years.

Children in the Stoke Mentoring programs have shown profound changes. The average high school graduation rate in New York City is sixty-five percent. Children in Stoke Mentoring have roughly a one hundred percent graduation rates. Children in this program become aware they can learn a skill, have fun, channel energy in a creative way, learn how to get up after falling, overcome obstacles, and achieve success. If I had had this program as a child, I might not have made the choices I made.

What I have learned has become what I aspire to teach. If you are dedicated to yourself, then you stay on the path; you keep using whatever clues you can to put the pieces back together, really self-actualize, and become the best version of yourself that you can be. Ultimately, that means serving other people in a way that is unique and fulfills both you and them.

COMMENTARY BY PAUL SCHIENBERG PhD

YOGA FOR ADDICTION RECOVERY

Jonathan had many traumatic moments in his youth. The death of his father, who he loved so very much, was the most crushing emotional experience. He turned to many substances in his attempts to solve his emotional anguish. He drank a great deal and ended up in a rehab.

There is a "bad" old joke that goes something like this:

Addicted Friend 1: Have you stopped using drugs and alcohol?

Addicted Friend 2: Oh yeah! Sure!

Addiction: 1: Really? That is great. How did you do it?

Addicted Friend 2: Stopping is not a problem. I've done it a thousand times.

This is a very typical "joke" told by many people who have struggled with addictions.

This was very true with Jonathan. He had stopped using many substances many times. This pattern repeated itself to the point where he was at a breaking point. Finally, he found a "medicine" that stuck and really turned him in the right direction permanently. It was a combination of twelve-step programs and yoga. He became completely dedicated to his daily yoga exercise, and he developed a yoga practice and helped many people conquer addiction.

YOGA AS MEDICINE

With relapse rates higher than 40 percent, addiction specialists and those in recovery are turning to adjunct therapies such as yoga. The goal is to give addicts the skills they need to learn to tolerate the uncomfortable feelings and sensations that can lead to relapse.

Yoga is highly effective at regulating stress hormones, including cortisol and adrenaline. These imbalances can lead to anxiety disorders, depressions, PTSD, and substance abuse. If yoga can help people maintain these hormone levels, there's a chance they won't feel the need to resort to substances to cope with these feelings.

Yoga is increasingly being used in substance abuse treatment programs and throughout recovery to help prevent relapse, reduce withdrawal symptoms and drug cravings, and provide a healthy outlet to cope with potential triggers and daily life stressors.

ADDICTION IS DIS-EASE AND YOGA BRINGS EASE

Addiction is a state of mind and body where we feel distant from ease. It is this lack of ease that compels a person to reach for something to try to feel better or move them closer to ease. Therefore, any practice that can bring ease to a body-mind system, which is productive rather than destructive, will be a key ingredient on the path to recovery from addiction. The physical practice of yoga, along with breath practices, serves to detoxify the body and to calm the mind. Yoga improves circulation and lung capacity, stretches and strengthens muscles, helps to work out the organs, improves digestion, and regulates the nervous and endocrine systems. A recovering addict will simply be more comfortable in his/her mind and body. Yoga is a central and necessary component of recovery from addiction.

EMPTINESS FUELS ADDICTION AND YOGA COUNTERS THIS

People who struggle with addiction carry a deep sense of lack. Something seems to be missing. An itch needs to be scratched. With acute addiction, one's entire organism is caught in a pursuit to fulfill needs that can never be met. This is true for active addicts as much as it is true for people in recovery—until they have been able to work out the complex roots of trauma that drives their behavior.

In the body's hierarchy of needs, breath is our highest. We can live without food for weeks. We can live without water for days. The way we breathe directly affects our emotional state, and our emotional state affects the way we breathe. When we feel anxious, worried, angry, or stressed, our breath becomes shallow. Interestingly, it sends a signal to our nervous system that our core need is not being met. This reinforces a sense of lack which creates tension and stress. For addicts, this is dangerous, because it keeps us stuck in a somatic pattern that reinforces the illusion that we are incomplete. It keeps us stuck in the force field of addiction.

The word "yoga" means union. It refers to the union of mind, body, and spirit. Yoga practice is the practice of connecting or re-connecting with my body. In active addiction, we have lost connection with our body. Addiction counters even our body's main directive, our mind; to bring us back into contact with our physical self will move us toward a sense of union and will be uplifting to our spirit.

THE LIFE ISSUES LIVE IN OUR TISSUES

Addiction has its roots in trauma, which I define as any event that leaves undigested or unprocessed negative emotional energy stuck in the mind-body system. Our biography becomes our biology. Among its benefits, Kundalini yoga helps to detoxify and rebuilt the systems of the body. It gets deep and can move energy, unlike any other thing some traumatized people have experienced.

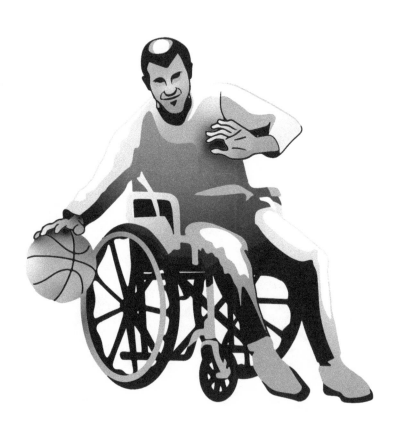

PART III

ACTIVITIES THAT GAVE US A SPORTING CHANCE AT LIFE

CHAPTER 12

BRIAN'S STORY: YOGA HEALS ME— BODY AND SOUL

"Yoga became my medicine. I did yoga during the day and twelve-step meetings in the evening. Both activities helped turn off that part of my brain that felt defective . . . I felt sane again."

MY FATHER WAS A chronic diabetic. He was in and out of the hospital and died when I was fourteen years old.

The loss of my father was not sudden. From ages four to fourteen, my father's illness was the centerpiece of my family life. It was a huge financial strain, and there were constant arguments about how to deal with his health and money.

I cared a great deal for my dad. In his later years, he became a stay-at-home parent, and we spent a lot of time together. My mother worked and kept the family financially afloat. I have a close relationship with her now, even though I didn't see much of her then. My dad's family, his sisters and brothers, all struggled with the disease and lost various body parts over time as a result. When I was in first grade, my father had lost a leg. By the sixth grade, my father had a major stroke, lost the other leg, and was in a wheelchair. In addition, my dad's mental capacity deteriorated. He began to disappear. I spent a lot of time in the hospital with him after school. The physical therapists, nurses, and doctors all knew me by name.

After my father's death, I was left with anger and depression about his dying and his absence. Why didn't he do what he needed to get better? My dad was not a great patient. He didn't exercise, diet, keep up regular visits with the doctor, or check his blood sugar levels. My father avoided doing anything that would have prolonged his life.

This horrible period was extremely hard on my mother as well. She was exhausted most of the time from work. Meanwhile, I developed an independent streak. And while I was a member of a large extended family, I always felt like I was observing everything from the outside. I coped by going into the bedroom, closing the door, reading books, and creating a fantasy world.

A DIAMOND AND COURT AT THE CENTER OF MY WORLD

Baseball was at the center of my sports world. My father had insisted on it. Originally, I didn't want to play, and cried all the way to the baseball field. I was afraid the other kids would pick on me. I stuck with it, though, and actually grew to really like playing baseball as my performance improved. Day after day, I would find myself on the field, practicing. It was like my oasis away from what was happening at home. I got into organized baseball and played two days a week.

I also learned to play tennis by seventh and eighth grade and really enjoyed it. Tennis was so much more physically engaging than baseball. It was a great workout and you only needed two people to play. Tennis required much more self-reliance and was physically and mentally demanding. There was more strategy and the game pitted one person against another. I loved that.

The years after age fourteen were very dark ones for me. I hung out with maybe one or two close friends, stayed indoors, and watched TV.

I worked hard to get very good grades, but there was no denying I was depressed. I got into Princeton after graduating high school and I was determined to thrive academically. I believed it was my only ticket out of the darkness—just like sports had been in my earlier years.

Then the past caught up with me. An incident that took place eighteen years ago started a major snowball effect. I had gone to a concert at Roseland with a group of three other friends to celebrate one of their birthdays. It was going to be a weekend bash. On the Saturday night of the concert, we raided one of our parents' liquor cabinets and drank a lot alcohol on the bus to Manhattan. My emotional pain disappeared as I drank and got high. All the pressure was gone. I don't remember much of that night other than sitting upstairs in a lounge and marveling at some fuzzy wallpaper.

I didn't go home that weekend—didn't even call. That was a big deal. From that weekend on, I continued to crave that freedom. I had found this external thing that was going to release me from what had felt like such a big burden for so long. Over the next several months, alcohol had become the centerpiece of all social interactions. All that mattered was how, where, and when I was going to get my hands on it.

A MAJOR IN ALCOHOLISM AT PRINCETON

I left for Princeton that September. It was a big uprooting. I had not set a foot in Princeton before, and now I was living there. I got dropped off and all I had was a bag of clothes, raging alcoholism, anger, sadness, and depression. It was much easier to get alcohol on the campus. Under the influence of alcohol, I stopped attending all the classes. In my first two years at Princeton, I probably attended about twenty classes. Regardless, I got a B average over those years.

By age twenty, I had been drinking for three years and added drugs to my attempts to self-medicate. I smoked marijuana, snorted cocaine, and took psychedelic drugs like LSD and mushrooms. In other words, I ingested anything that gave me a different psychological feeling.

It was becoming harder for me to string two coherent thoughts together. I started to have delusional thoughts. Though these thoughts were not destructive, my behavior was, and I realized that I needed help.

I was terrified. One day, over a cup of coffee, a female friend convinced me that alcohol and drugs were causing most, if not all, of my problems. She knew someone who was part owner of a rehab program in Florida, and she set up a meeting for me. That meeting, six weeks before the end of the school year, completely changed my life.

The owner offered me a free spot in the rehab center if I could get a plane ticket. I was skeptical and really scared. I wasn't sure that I wanted to give up alcohol and drugs. But the owner stuck with me and kept urging me to come to the rehab. Finally, I gave in and went to Florida to spend six weeks as an in-patient.

I stayed another six weeks after that, too. During the additional six weeks, the owner offered me a place to stay in return for my doing some landscaping and other odd jobs during this period. In just twelve weeks, this man saved my life.

OPRAH INTRODUCES ME TO LIFE-SAVING YOGA

It's been almost sixteen years of sobriety for me. But even though I was alcohol and drug free, all the internal stuff that pushed me to use was still to be dealt with. There were some dark days still ahead of me.

At the rehab center, I was introduced to the practice of yoga, but not in the usual way. One day during Fourth of July weekend, when all the activities were cancelled, I was sitting around with nothing to do. I felt really depressed being so far from home and having nothing to look forward to, till I turned on the Oprah Winfrey show. She had a yoga teacher as a guest who asked the audience to stand up and do yoga. She showed the audience four or five different poses, and I did them along with the audience. After finishing the segment, I didn't want to get back on the couch. Instead, I went to the training room. I began to run on the treadmill and found all this new energy that I hadn't experienced before. I made a commitment to myself that day; I would keep moving. I got up every day and did yoga on my own. I made notes about the different poses that I did every day. It made a huge difference in my well-being. I didn't fall into depression again during my stay at the rehab in Florida.

When I returned to the same environment where I had been abusing, I saw the same people I drank and did drugs with. Now I was faced with another big question—what was I going to do with my life? I found a yoga class at a gym, signed up, and started going twice a week. I didn't skip one class. Yoga became my medicine. I did yoga during the day and twelve-step meetings in the evening. Both activities helped turn off that part of my brain that felt defective. The positive effect lasted longer and longer.

I FELT SANE AGAIN.

I got a job in marketing that lasted about seven years and continued my yoga practice during this time. Then when my dedication to my yoga practice began to slip away, I thought I was doing okay, but I was setting the stage to get into trouble again.

I was now twenty-six years old, with two friends in a car in Philadelphia. It was an icy night, and we got rear-ended by a taxi. There was no damage to the car, so the taxi and the car went their separate ways. I felt fine. But the next morning, I woke up and my back felt strange. It hurt to sit for a long period of time and my range of motion was different. I didn't seek medical attention, and over the next few weeks, it didn't go away. Instead, it got worse. Three weeks after the accident, I had excruciating pain going down both legs. I had difficulty sleeping. I couldn't sneeze without pain. The results of an MRI showed I had a degenerative disc disease. The cushioning between the vertebras that helped protect the nerves had worn away. Two of my discs had ruptured because of the car accident.

An orthopedist told me to start physical therapy and not do yoga again. I was in disbelief. I told myself that no one was going to tell me never to do yoga again. But I took the doctor's advice and did PT for three months. The pain subsided, but still there was a constant discomfort. When the insurance ran out, I was "thrown to the wolves." The doctor left me with instructions to ice it when it felt bad and take steroids. Instead, I went back to yoga. The pain became huge again—a major setback.

I stopped the yoga and re-entered physical therapy, using steroids and traction machines. While doing the physical therapy again, I noticed that many of the movements were similar to the poses of yoga. For example, when they asked me to stretch out on the floor on my belly, it was the same as the cobra pose in yoga. They were telling me not to do yoga and to do yoga at the same time.

BACK TO THE MAT FOR HEALING MYSELF AND OTHERS

I wanted to find a yoga class that was not just good for exercise, but also good for healing, for it had become clear that the mental and spiritual aspects of yoga could be helpful to me again—as they had been when I was in rehab. I was very lucky to find a yoga studio run by a chiropractor whose approach incorporated an attention to anatomical detail.

IT FELT LIKE MAGIC.

It was all that I wanted yoga to be—spiritual, mental, and physical. It shifted what I wanted to do with my life as it became clear that I wanted to do this for a living. I wanted to help people. I saw a lot of unnecessary suffering—physical, mental, and emotional—and I wanted to be part of a proactive solution for people who are dealing with pain and suffering.

So, I went on to get certified, because I wanted to teach. My first teaching gig was at a women's health center. I fell in love with it right away. I began to teach at a couple of studios. I created a website and started giving private lessons over the years. Today, I work with people who have either experienced an injury or have long-term pain, have had surgery, and so on. I customize the yoga teaching to each person's individual issues, and I have added massage therapy to my teaching tools. Along the way, I have acquired a lot of anatomical information. Not only do I design the daily yoga practice as it helps clients with their problems, but I also design the practice daily, depending on how he or she feels that day.

I have found my purpose through yoga—my calling. Utilizing its practice, I was able to find myself again. Not only have I healed myself, but I am also now blessed with the privilege of healing others.

COMMENTARY BY PAUL SCHIENBERG PhD

YOGA HEALS ME, BODY AND SOUL

Brian was angry at his father for not taking care of himself. His father and mother were not role models for how to take care of yourself.

Regardless of his success at sports and good grades, he was depressed. He got into Princeton which he hoped would be his way out of his darkness. It didn't work out that way because of a car accident.

That September, he entered Princeton. He attended very few of his classes even though he maintained a B average. By the time he reached twenty years old, he not only drank but was using marijuana, cocaine, LSD, and mushrooms. He took anything he could get to change his psychological state. He could barely talk coherently. He had become delusional.

A female friend of Brian's knew someone who was part owner of a rehab in Florida. That meeting between Brian and the co-owner changed his life. The owner was ongoingly pushing Brian to come to his rehab. Finally, Brian gave in and spent six weeks there for free. This began many years of substance abstinence. But the darkness and pain underneath had not been dealt with. There were many dark days left ahead of him. The memories of what happened didn't completely disappear and resurfaced in the years ahead. These events are common with people who have gone through painful experiences. They get triggered by events in the present.

At the rehab, Brian was introduced to yoga. It was July 4th and he turned on the Oprah Winfrey show. Her guest was a yoga instructor who was demonstrating many yoga poses. He followed along and the next day went to the training room at a gym and signed up and started going twice a week. So, yoga helped him turn off that part of his brain that he thought was defective.

His physical pain returned after another car accident. He went to a physical therapist. Brian realized that many of the movements that the physical therapists was doing with him were like yoga poses. So, Brian went in search of a yoga class that not only was good exercise but also helped with the pain. A yoga instructor who was also a chiropractor ran a class that attended to anatomical detail. He had found what he wanted to do with his life; combining physical, mental, and emotional yoga teaching became his life goal. He found his life purpose.

CHAPTER 13

HANK'S STORY: PREPARED FOR THE GAME BY THE SISTERS OF PERPETUAL PAIN

"Athletics gave me the self-worth to fulfill all these dreams. During the toughest times, sports pulled me through."

I SAT AT THE dining room table crying, my hands holding my head as upright as possible.

I was crying inside, as well. Shouting for help.

I couldn't live without alcohol. And I knew it was killing me. I was blacking out more frequently, and my life was taking a turn that might wind me up either in jail or dead. I was drinking on the job, and also before participating in athletic games, which I had never done before. Worse, I was also operating my truck while intoxicated. Before, I was always able to cover my drinking binges so they wouldn't interfere with my responsibilities.

Months ago, while I was driving my vehicle in my hometown, I got stopped by a police sergeant who knew me. He pulled me over, saying, "Hank, what the hell are you doing? Don't move. Stay right there. Sleep it off. If I find you on the road, I'm going to shoot you!" I did sleep it off that night. After that incident, I often let my older son—a fourteen-year–old—drive my truck because I was too inebriated to drive. Why was I doing this to him, to my wife, and to myself?

In desperation, I reached for the phone. Who could I call? I thought of Ray, a recovering alcoholic. I called him for help once ten years ago, but never followed through. Now I reached for the telephone, and he answered. "Ray," I cried, "I need help. I need to get sober."

"If you really mean it and want help," Ray said, "then meet me at the Congregational Church in New Milford at 7 P.M. tonight." I hung up the phone and immediately felt relief. Maybe I could just turn my life around. Maybe I could beat the booze.

BLUE COLLARS AND DIAMONDS

I was born in the Bronx in a blue-collar household. When I was about three months old, we relocated to Massachusetts, where Dad managed a dairy farm and Mom ran a boarding house. When I was six or seven, at the time when American troops left for the Korean War, we moved again to Danbury, Connecticut, where my parents worked in a defense plant. We had very little money at the time. I felt extremely self-conscious about our economic situation.

I was the youngest son, so it was my older "pain-in-the-butt" brother who took charge at home, since Mom and Dad got home later in the evening. I felt my brother sometimes acted aggressively toward me, and since I was a sensitive youngster, I saw it as bullying and was affected by it, especially after school, alone with him, when I wanted to play ball rather than do homework.

My parents, who were very Irish Catholic, sent me to parochial school rather than the public school most of my friends attended. I was not a good student, since I was more interested in sports and being outdoors. While hypersensitive and shy by nature, there was also a mischievous side to me—a rebellious lad who often defied the Catholic school authorities and their rules. I felt I didn't fit into their model of who I was meant to be, even nicknaming the nuns "Sisters of Perpetual Pain," since I felt they tortured youngsters. Since my school was five miles away, I was not a part of the neighborhood clique, and when I was in the sixth grade, the school resorted to double sessions to accommodate the growing student enrollment. My school day then began in the afternoon, so when I would normally be playing, I was either on my bike or on a school bus, and then there was homework, so I never could play baseball or basketball during the week.

To top it off, I began having anxiety attacks. For some unknown reason, I feared Mom dying and leaving me. I began having stomach problems as a result of these panic outbreaks, until our family doctor sent me to a pediatrician who addressed them.

He was my savior. "What Hank needs is to attend public school!" he said. "He is so removed from the local kids. He needs friends to play ball with after school. He needs to feel less isolated!" What an accurate diagnosis and prescription—a pediatrician ahead of his time! My parents listened and registered me in public middle school, where puberty took over.

I was captivated by the girls! I wanted to impress them and stand out. So, I started playing organized sports such as junior league baseball— sandlot baseball. It became a real passion.

I took to organized sports so quickly; I was so skillful that by seventh grade baseball and basketball became the remedies for my physical and emotional illnesses. I made friends, and instead of feeling segregated, I became one of the gangs. I changed dramatically from a shy, embarrassed young man to a more confident teen. I no longer focused on my parent's financial position; my self-worth was not dependent on their economic state. My self-esteem emanated from positive thoughts of excelling—win or die—in sports!

SAVED BY SPORT FOR THE FIRST TIME

For the first time, sports were making an impact in my life. I was a valuable player on the team and other kids looked up to me. Even the pretty cheerleaders wanted to cheer my name at games. Being part of a team—this new "sports figure" role—gave me more self-assurance and freedom. My life revolved around staying eligible for sports by getting passing grades. It was a tough time for me because I was always on the verge of failing. I had no trouble when it came to physical education (of course!), social studies, or world history, but the other subjects were not only difficult for me, but I had no interest in them. So, I struggled to stay afloat until I reached high school.

My older brother attended a technical high school, where he played basketball. I had no idea that the tech school would be interested in my enrolling. But they were. I had never thought about college as an option for me, for financial reasons, but Abbott Tech offered classes like machine shop, provided I studied some regular academic subjects as well. The teachers at Abbott treated us like adults as they prepared us for jobs in industry.

I was on the Abbott varsity squad for four years and went to the state quarter finals in my first year. I was always in the local newspapers and on local TV for winning tournaments! I was a star. I was a hot shot!

Now that I was a big shot, I started acting like one. I had friends older than me who looked up to me—a fifteen-year-old! So, for fun, we would drive from Danbury to nearby Brewster, New York, to a bar on Putnam Lake. Drinking age was eighteen in New York at the time, and just a little swig gave me such a buzz, I felt I could do anything. No longer was that underlying feeling nagging me that maybe—just maybe—I wasn't that good an athlete, a feeling I was familiar with otherwise, even though I was revered as a star. And, while I loved girls, I still had a little shyness around them. Abbott Tech was an all-boys school, so meeting girls wasn't always easy, with no sororities and fraternities bonding us. Our tech school was often viewed as a "hood school," where you learn a trade, no college prep. So here I was, a celebrity; my face was on every front page of the newspaper, and I still had trouble talking to girls. I fit in on the outside, but inside, I was still left out.

MY EGO, THE BIGGEST LOSER!

When I was in my senior year, my parents were working in a factory in Bethel, Connecticut, and one day Dad's boss asked if I had received any offers for college. Since college was the furthest thing from my mind, I had no thoughts about applying. But Dad came home and told me his boss had gone to Iona College and wanted to introduce me to the basketball coach there.

Dad's boss took me to Iona and, after an interview, I was offered a full four-year basketball scholarship! The only caveat was that I had to pass the college boards within the next month. I took the exams and passed math but not English. Iona really wanted me, though, so they set up tutoring sessions for me during the summer and even paid for the tutor. But I copped an attitude. "If Iona really wants me, they'll make an exception." But they didn't. My unexpected opportunity to play college basketball was stymied by my "I do not need to comply by your rules" attitude. Now what?

Out of school, I toyed with the idea of going into the Navy. Funny I should think about that as a career. Though I had copped a "star" attitude with Iona College, I sure couldn't cop one with the Navy! So, with that idea on the back burner, I went from star to soda jerk. It was summer and I worked at a drive-in restaurant where I met Loretta. The good thing was that I met lots of girls; the bad thing is that I continued to write my story of failure as I beat myself up for not being worthy, not a good enough ball player. I took another part-time job at an A&P in the meat department. There I got quite an education from the older employees. They liked to party! After work, a group of us would go out drinking with sorority girls. To live up to my own expectations, I had to drink and *drink*. Liquor led me.

I continued playing baseball for pick-up teams in the summer from May to July, and coached industrial adult leagues. I even started refereeing for city league teams. Basketball didn't start until fall. All this time, I dated and drank. And I continued to see Loretta.

I liked my part-time job at the A&P. I would have liked a full-time job there, but there were no opportunities, so I got a job at a Safeway meat department. And after work, I went out till 3 or 4 A.M. and back into work at 8 A.M., until I got laid off.

IN THE NAVY NOW

I found out that the captain of our Bethel team was going in to talk with a Navy recruiter and I went along. Though my friend told him we were looking for the Navy recruiter, this Marine was going for the full salesmanship job. He pulled out all the stops and almost convinced us to go into the Marines! But then the Navy officer appeared and we naively—without thinking too much about the consequences—signed up on the spot. When I told Mom what I had done, she freaked out, though Dad was in the Navy, so what was the problem? I would go to boot camp, take an aptitude test, and get a school guaranteed rating as an engine or radar man. My girlfriend Loretta said she would wait for me. Not bad!

I took the aptitude test, hoping to get a job as a cook like Dad, but I scored high on the exam for a radio man, which meant radio school. Boot camp was a breeze for me because we played sports. Other enlistees had such trouble at boot camp—crying because the discipline and games was too much for them. But remember, I was used to the Sisters of the Presentation of Pain!

I was such a good student in radio school. I held a 4.0 and no less than a 3.8 or 3.9 for my grade averages. Succeeding as a student changed my whole outlook on studying. I had to do well. But I didn't do well in the booze area.

After boot camp, I blacked out on vodka at a New Year's Eve party. I thought I was functioning okay, but apparently I was doing weird stuff. Afterwards, I felt real shame. So, I vowed never to drink vodka again.

As a radio man for the Navy, I progressed in rank to an E4. I applied for security clearance—the highest one—in top secret decoding during the Cuban Missile Crisis. True to form, that nagging voice reappeared, telling me, "I'm going to screw up." I didn't screw up at that or in playing organized sports for the Navy—including the All-Navy Tournament we played at colleges in Virginia. But while I did well in sports, the responsibility I felt in holding this top-secret position was intense and set a tone. Drinking became an important part of my Navy life.

During my third year in the Navy, I became engaged to Loretta, but after once again blacking out, I broke off the engagement because I couldn't handle the responsibility. We got back together again, and when Loretta told me she was pregnant, we eloped and got married in North Carolina. I was twenty-two years old, and Loretta was under twenty-one.

We set up in Norfolk, Virginia, where I was assigned to the shore communications station. I worked the day shift from seven in the morning until three in the afternoon. We lived in a small cottage where I continued to drink, feeling I had things under control. We didn't have a lot of money, and whatever extra I had, I used to buy booze.

One afternoon, I came home to find Loretta crying, doubled over, having been in pain from cramps all day. The baby was coming. We had to get to the Navy hospital. But Loretta, in bed, could not be moved. I contacted a crewman who was trained as an EMT, and he came just in time. I caught baby Scott, and then called the emergency number to take mom and babe to the hospital.

My enlistment was almost up. The US was involved now in the Vietnam War. I wanted to re-up and make a career out of the Navy. Radiomen were going to Southeast Asia. Loretta wasn't happy about this decision, to say the least, and she made it clear. So that wasn't going to happen.

WHEN EVEN SPORTS FAIL TO SAVE

I met a friend from high school while I was looking for a job and we were living with my parents. He mentioned that the phone company was hiring and that my radioman skills could be transferred to a position as an installer-repairman. I was hired. You would think that I would fully embrace this new opportunity to finally be more responsible, but no, my drinking started to pick up. I felt such enormous accountability—house, family, job—that I began to have the old panic attacks. I knew I couldn't drink on the job, but my heart raced as the anxiety worsened.

I decided to seek treatment from a doctor who diagnosed anxiety and prescribed tranquilizers, which worked. But one day on the job when I felt that panicky feeling and reached for a sedative, one of the workers saw me and said, "That stuffs for women. Meet me after work and I will show you how to relax." I quickly learned that evening how to take the edge off—a shot of rye and a glass of beer. My old friend booze helped make me loosen up and act with self-confidence. Rye and beer were now my new medications, and I was once again living life in the lap of liquor.

I drank daily—a six-pack, flavored brandy, whatever took the edge off. I seemed to have more freedom to drink on the job, and had it under control, at least I thought. I didn't have too many blackouts.

My wife didn't work, and though I was making good money, bills and other household expenses piled up, and now a second son was on the way. I kept telling myself to drink less, to slow down, just drink to get through the anxiety. But I couldn't slow down.

I was still playing ball in adult leagues, and I drank, but always later, never during a game. I was still playing well and winning some championships. I even played against Marques Haynes, a basketball great, and his Harlem Globetrotters.

Whatever I did, drinking became a part of it. When I fished, I carried beer along. Hangovers were more frequent, so on Mondays, I began calling in sick to work. I drank more and more to prolong the *buzz* feeling. This was the vicious cycle of panic and booze.

Then I began drinking before games. Athletics and sports had been my way out of panic, my way to shine. Instead, baseball and basketball no longer pulled me out of my rut. I started having the shakes and drinking on the job became normal. I couldn't live without alcohol. I was being questioned at work. Why was I always calling in sick on Mondays? The boss confronted me with the fact that I had called out because of the flu six times. So what was going on?

And then there was that life-changing night at the kitchen table when I realized I had to get help and Ray told me to meet him at the Congregational Church, saying, "Try not to drink, Hank. Just meet me there."

I went to my first AA meeting on April 7, 1980. I have not had to pick up a drink since. By the way, my granddaughter was born on that date twenty-four years later. That night more than ever, I realized I still needed a reason to stay sober. I was thirty-eight years old and still playing basketball and softball, but it just wasn't enough. I thought about the fact that my older son raced motocross, and I had often thought to myself, *When I'm sober, I'll try motocross, to focus my energy into racing to fill the void.*

I did just that, focusing on maintaining my bike, as I was gaining sobriety, I took to that bike just as I did to baseball and basketball. Within four years, I was number one!

I was too old to play ball, but I was not too old to race motocross in the spring and fall. In the winter, I enjoyed ice races, which were a lot of fun. I even began fishing again, this time without the beer.

After my first year of sobriety, my wife started drinking heavily. She said, "Hank, I've put up with you all these years. You will have to put up with me now." But I couldn't, and we divorced. Eventually, the boys, ages fifteen and twelve, both wanted to stay with me.

Soon our lives were filled with this new sport—a most demanding one. You need physical conditioning to race motocross. I was forty-seven or forty-eight years old, still with the phone company, but now a better employee. I was offered a promotion as a manager. Though someone else got that job, the fact that I was offered the position and tried for it was what counted.

I excelled on the job and in sport, which kept me sober. I raced in Daytona on professional tracks. I qualified for national competitions at the Foxboro Stadium in Massachusetts. Only when I injured my knee did I question how long I could continue motocross. After all, the jumps were increasingly demanding. I knew I couldn't go pro at my age and with my knee injury. It was time to give it up, so I hung up my helmet after ten years. Now what?

NOTHING HAPPENS BY ACCIDENT

One day my youngest son went on a skiing trip with his girlfriend. They got stuck in a snowstorm, and their car had to be towed. They rented a condo and I drove up to be with them. Since their car was not going to be ready to be returned until the next day, I was stuck there for the night and possibly the next day. The next morning, the kids went skiing. What was I going to do with myself? I walked out of the condo to the slopes and there I saw a ski package—lesson, ski rental, gear and group lesson to start at 11 A.M. I bought the package. I remember getting on the ski lift and doing parallel turns before the lesson even began. And the bug bit me! I was hooked! I loved skiing so much and skied so often that, within four years, I became a ski instructor. This is where I belonged. This is my sport.

It is interesting what paths our lives take and how they cross. When I was a kid, I dreamed of teaching physical education and going into law enforcement. I have taught skiing—which, to me, is physical education—to over 2,000 kids over a twenty-year span. I have taught kids and their kids. Now I have the pleasure to teach skiing in the winter and, ten years ago, I had an opportunity to take a job for the summer in Washington, Connecticut, at a boat launch, riding on the water, inspecting the water for infestation. I do Lake Patrol with a police officer, promoting safety—a kind of law enforcement job.

Dreams are just dreams unless they are fulfilled. My void is certainly overflowing. Years ago, I became a first responder, an EMT. I get paid to do what I love, and I've been blessed to have saved a couple lives and comfort many people through these years.

Athletics gave me the self-worth to fulfill all these dreams. During the toughest times, sports pulled me through. The thing, though, that made everything possible was that phone call to Ray saying I needed to do something about my drinking. I wouldn't be alive today and certainly would never have touched the lives of others if it hadn't been for Ray and my love of sports. I have received accolades, awards, trophies, and lots of recognition for my contribution to sports and my athletic abilities, but if it that phone call hadn't happened, my life would have been empty.

I'm seventy-two now.

Maybe it's time to play golf!

COMMENTARY BY MARILYN GANSEL PsyD

WHAT ARE SELF-DESTRUCTIVE BEHAVIORS?

Self-destructive behaviors are harmful actions toward oneself. An extreme result of self-destruction would be suicide. These actions are sometimes intentional, like cutting oneself or engaging in reckless behavior such as going on a hunger strike. Self-destructive patterns provide a coping mechanism to deal with emotional turmoil. At the root of this behavior is childhood trauma.

All of us act from time to time as if we are in a self-destructive mode. But when the behavior is extreme and habitual with loss of control, then that behavior alleviates a painful memory—a past story the person remembers and believes is real about him or her. It is that person's mechanism for avoiding their true feelings. They may also use this self-injurious behavior to punish themselves or provide some relief or pleasure that is short-term; life for that person is never fulfilling or satisfying.

ORIGINS

Youngsters who view themselves as poor, self-conscious, and sensitive can find themselves rebellious. They often don't fit the story of who they are supposed to be by societal norms. Their exterior persona reflecting destructive behaviors create psychological problems like anxiety and physical concerns like stomach issues. So it was only when Hank articulated the origin of his persistent and destructive behaviors that he was able to slowly gain control over his impulses. He needed to become aware of the formative years that shaped the story of who he believed he was.

CHANGE YOUR STORY

It is never too late to rewrite your story. Choosing a new way of believing despite parental upbringing—or ingrained negative messages or school pressures—takes effort and work. Like an athlete, it needs practice, visualization, and a change of mindset. It requires experimenting with different support systems that open the door to meaning, purpose, and fulfillment. Those support systems increase proficiencies that help boost self-confidence. Even mistakes we make along our journey teach us to find opportunities to learn and grow. So, participating in organized sport, for example, releases physical and emotional distress. Sport becomes the vehicle that allows individuals to showcase their abilities and feel competent. Sport pushes the nagging voice inside your mind that says you aren't enough to go away. Sport helps a team of young athletes develop resilience to move forward in a healthy, responsible manner.

PRESSURE ON

The nagging voice inside Hank's head that told him he will "screw up" on the field or he wasn't really a "good athlete" further added to his negative sense of self. His old story of failure played over again in his mind. This set the stage for Hank's dependence on alcohol to relax and feel self-confident. Later came responsibilities to a job and wife and with it the need to drink without regard for his well-being or how it affected others around him. Liquor led him.

INTERVENTION AND REDEMPTION

It is said that we sometimes must hit bottom to seek recovery or ask for help. In Hank's case, phoning his friend Ray changed his story of failure to victory. What is interesting is what Hank chose to replace his addictive and self-destructive behavior—motocross! An outdoor physical activity! Added to his newfound activity was fishing and skiing. Those interests gave him a sporting chance at life. As Hank learned, sports play such a positive role in supporting mental health. For him, it opened doors to discover new hobbies at each stage of his life without the old self-destructive behavior—drinking to excess.

CHAPTER 14

OUR PERSONAL RESILIENCY STORIES:

MY MOUNTAIN TO CLIMB
Written by Paul Schienberg, PhD

OOOOPS! SOMETHING WENT WRONG when I was born. Very wrong. My digestive system was fine at its beginning, but not at its end. That was the problem; my intestines ended abruptly, instead of there being an opening. Elimination was impossible.

To come into the world with this birth defect was very rare and extremely dangerous.

CALLING ALL HEROES

It was 1947, a dramatic year for Jackie Robinson and me. Later I would become Jackie's biggest fan. When the rest of my friends were rooting for Yankees like Whitey Ford, Joe DiMaggio, and Mickey Mantle, I was the only kid rooting for that nonwhite guy playing for the Dodgers. Jackie Robinson—and then Don Newcombe, Roy Campanella, Joe Black, and Junior Gilliam—became my powerful examples of underdogs who overcame, who seemed to have undying hope, unlimited strength, fierce courage, and determination.

My condition required all the heroes I could find. My situation was not only life-threatening, but often humiliating. The first day of my life involved surgery—a colostomy. I was in such trouble that my parents could have chosen to let me go. Instead, they opted for more surgeries, hoping to get me to normalcy.

My mother began to research pediatric surgeons who knew of this defect and had a belief that they could be of help. She finally found Dr. Swenson, the needle in the haystack.

THE BODY NEVER FORGETS

Finally, after many surgeries with Dr. Swenson at Boston Floating Hospital, he created the biological piece that had been missing. I endured fourteen surgeries in seven years. Some of the surgeries were successful, and a few created other problems. Regardless, I finally reached an important physical milestone, and I am grateful for it.

Half of my surgeries occurred before I developed the ability to speak. Therefore, my conscious memory of those necessary early operations is not accessible to me. I would learn later that those traumatic experiences were embedded in my neurology, bones, muscles, anxieties, and so on. I didn't revisit those places until years later. There were the scars reminding me each day that there had been many attacks upon my body. I would experience intestinal obstructions caused by internal scar tissue, and even flashes of partial visual memories, all hints of what had occurred in those early years.

The largest physical and psychological problems I faced were connected to the fact that it would take me ten more years before I would develop sphincter control of my bowels. During this period, I had many embarrassing accidents that left deep emotional scarring.

I was angry at my body. I was extremely depressed and felt like a freak. I did not know anyone who had this problem. My body was out of control. I struggled with shame, jealousy, isolation, and hopelessness. I had no one to talk to about these feelings. It was the 1950s, when it did not occur to anyone to think of seeing a therapist.

A BODY I COULD NEVER TRUST

The only place of safety I had was my family home. School was a place of terror. At any moment, I might have a problem and be sent home. Everyone knew. My fellow students would make fun of me. I was not bullied, exactly, but I was laughed at and called names. They were angry at me stinking up their class. But the next day, I would be sent off to school to face the same students again.

I couldn't even depend on my own body.

I was also very angry at my parents for making me go back to school to face the scene of my "crime." It was a powerless and agonizing period of my young life. And I felt as though it would never end.

My parents would not allow me to completely withdraw into the shell I wanted to crawl into. At times, I remember hating them for it. After school, they would tell me to go to the playground, one block away from my home. It had a baseball field, four basketball and handball courts, and football field lines drawn on the cement.

I was a scrawny kid. Most of the children were built normally. They had sports equipment that included baseball bats and gloves, softballs, and basketballs. I did not have any of those items. The young kids would make two teams. I would watch them choose the best to the worst athletes, take the field, and play the game while I sat on the bench. This went on for many weeks, weekday after weekday, and weekend after weekend. I loved watching them play but could not imagine being picked.

THE LOUDEST APPLAUSE I EVER HEARD

One cloudy Saturday, there were not enough kids to fill out one of the teams. I watched as every kid was picked, leaving one team short; they needed a right fielder. "Hey, you. Want to play?" The captain of one of the teams pointed at me. "Sure. But I don't have a glove." One of the other team's players offered me his glove while he was at bat. I was so scared. Secretly, I prayed no one would hit the ball to me. They didn't.

It was the third inning before I got up to bat, and I was just hoping to contact the ball.

I did, and it flew in between the two outfielders! It was the greatest experience of my young life. I could run fast, so I ended up at third. The kids on my team were clapping and I was smiling, even though I tried to be cool about it. My body had worked, and it gave me pleasure.

I BELONGED!

My isolation was gone—at least for that day. I was one of the guys. I was part of a team. The rest of that summer was filled with playing baseball. I got picked every week to be part of one of the teams. "He's fast. He can hit. Pick him." These were lyrics I could not have been happier to hear.

At the end of this wonderful summer, I begged my father to help me buy a baseball glove, a hardball, and a bat. He was willing to take me to a sporting goods store to select a mitt. The leather of the glove smelled so sweet, and its signature was Carl Furillo, the right fielder for the Brooklyn Dodgers. My dad threw a can of leather oil into the shopping bag. When we got home, I oiled the mitt, stuck the baseball in it, folded it closed, and wrapped it very tightly with rope. I was thus equipped to move further into the world, and felt a sense of belonging, legitimacy. The only times I would unwrap the glove that fall was when I watched a left-handed pitcher throw on TV. You see, I am left-handed. I would spend hours modeling the form of pitchers like Whitey Ford and Sandy Koufax.

MY BODY AND I ON THE SAME TEAM

Somehow, I coaxed my parents into letting me join the Little League the next year. When my father called someone at the league, he found out there was no spot left for me unless he was willing to coach a team. He agreed, and I was thrilled beyond description. I spent the winter preparing myself by improving my running, throwing, and catching. I was gaining a sense of competency by getting my body to do what I wanted it to do.

My identity was changing and shifting at the same time. I felt that I could learn and develop—not just physically—socially as well.

Years later, I would read a book written by Sigmund Freud. He noted that our relationship with our body was the foundation for our mastery of every stage of our psychological and social development. If we have had a bad relationship with our body, it would create emotional anguish and interfere with achieving many life goals. I had a terrible relationship with my body until that wonderful summer when my body became my ally for the first time, and I promised myself that I would do what I could to take care of it.

When the next spring rolled around and it was the start of the Little League season, I got my first uniform—cap (blue), jersey with the number 3 on the back (Billy Cox of the Brooklyn Dodgers wore number 3), leggings, and pants. I was told to report to a spot on the baseball diamond where fifteen guys—all wearing blue—were gathered. I was welcomed by my teammates for that summer. What a great feeling. I belonged and we would be sharing the summer together—cheering, yelling, crying, connecting, and playing the game.

I pitched and played first base. Making the All-Star Team was the icing on the cake. I was not a great player, but I was good enough to belong and contribute to my team.

SPORT NEVER CEASES TO HEAL

Life was far from perfect after that summer. I have had intestinal obstructions a few times a year. After each episode, I was psychologically depleted and depressed. I needed to rebuild my sense of confidence in my body. So, I would go to the golf driving range, the batting cage, or I would swim or run. It was always like starting all over again. But, this treatment worked, and soon I would find myself feeling my confidence coming back.

Over my desk, I have signed photographs of Don Newcombe, Carl Furillo, Johnny Podres, Preacher Roe, Roy Campanella, and Billy Loes. Those men who played for the Brooklyn Dodgers were a very important piece of the puzzle for me, showing me how to find myself and live a life filled with hope, achievements, and a sense of belonging. Sport has been and will always be a part of my life.

Life has its up and downs. It can throw us in all directions at a moment's notice. Many events are neither predictable nor controllable. No one escapes these experiences without being profoundly affected. It takes flexibility, skill, confidence, courage, and a belief in yourself to overcome them. Participation in sports and exercise can help build those characteristics that will serve us in climbing these mountains throughout our lives.

NO END TO THE MOUNTAINTOPS

Some of these challenges were imposed upon us by biology. I remember when I volunteered for the Special Olympics in Los Angeles, helping mentally and physically impaired children train to perform in various sports. The experience was so moving. The smiles on their faces were remarkable as they grew into athletes competing against other much challenged children. You could see their pride and confidence shining through. One of those children came up to me after noticing the scars on my abdomen. Without hesitating, he said, "That must have hurt." We bonded immediately and I spent the rest of my day watching him climb his mountain.

Other mountains are made up of the impact of abuse that some suffered from others—verbally and physically. Sometimes the verbal mountains are even harder to overcome than biological challenges. Why? The scars were not physical and therefore other people had more difficulty appreciating their impact. The mountains they created were made of feelings of worthlessness, lack of trust, or wanting to be hurt again. So, those kids became isolated. Team sports are such a great way to climb that mountain.

Prejudice has been another creator of challenges. For athletes like Jesse Owens, Mohammad Ali, Jackie Robinson, Billie Jean King, and many others, sport and exercise became the method they used to climb their mountains.

One day, not long ago, I decided I wanted to get to the top of the highest mountain in Europe—Mount Blanc. It sits on the corner of Italy, France, and Switzerland, 14,000 feet high. I started one summer day, and seven days later, I was at the top. Looking back on those wonderful days, I realized that conquering this mountain was one of the great achievements of my life.

I had come to trust myself and feel confident that I could climb any mountain. I knew there would be more mountains to climb, for life is filled with them.

The beginning of the climb was my participation in the everyday miracles of sport and exercise.

CHAPTER 15

OUR PERSONAL RESILIENCY STORIES:

MORE THAN A FIFTY-POUND WEIGHT WAS LIFTED

Written by Marilyn Gansel, PsyD

I HIT ROCK BOTTOM after our daughter was born. Our daughter could not digest cow's milk; projectile-vomiting occurred every several hours. As a colicky baby, our little girl was a handful. I was still recovering from my C-section and had little patience—probably because I was so tired. I did not return to work for three months as I wanted to spend time with our baby, and I needed to take care of me. What I began to realize was, while motherhood was what I wanted, I now felt extremely isolated. I missed my work, my daily interactions with faculty, students, and parents. I became bored at home. I tried to fill up the time with home tasks; Martha Stewart would have been proud. I baked bread, prepared homemade baby food, painted rooms, and performed all the daily household tasks. Once, tired of the old, yellow-stained wall-to-wall carpeting in our living and dining rooms, I even tore them up, leaving the tacks around the perimeter of the rooms. Dumping the rolled carpet in the driveway, I waited for my husband to congratulate me on a job well done. Unfortunately, he did not think that was a job for which I was to be commended. All these tasks kept me busy but not fulfilled.

My husband took an early morning newspaper route to help us

financially. It was sad to see him waken around 3 A.M. and leave in rain and snow—all kinds of weather—to deliver newspapers in the wealthier sections of Greenwich, CT. I remember standing at the window with our daughter in my arms, waving to him as he drove out the driveway. Then he would return by 7 A.M. to shower and leave for his full-time job. It was a hard time for us. But it got harder still.

When my maternity leave was up, I returned to my teaching job. Every morning before school began, I would pack up our daughter and bring her to the babysitter's home where she played with other children. Then I would high-tail it to work. My life was running from home to sitter to work to sitter to home to university. I never stopping racing through my day and night. I was delighted to be back to work, although I didn't realize just how exhausting this routine could be. I had also decided to pursue a master's degree in library science which started evenings at a university at least a forty-five-minute one-way commute. It was a challenging time for me to balance everything, even though my husband supported me fully by taking care of our girl in the evenings so I could focus on my studies.

And then one morning, I was getting out of the shower. I bent over to put one leg into my panties, and I fell on my face. I couldn't move. I experienced such excruciating pain in my back. My husband got me to a doctor, but the pain was so unbearable; sciatic pain shot down my legs so I could not perform any daily tasks. I was ordered to bed; for a time, I lived at my parents' home. They took care of our daughter and me. During that period—the running part of my life, the time I chose to be even more "perfect" to prove myself to the world—I was beginning to experience insomnia. I could not fall asleep, or if I did, I would wake up at 3 or 4 in the morning and think, *I must go to work*. My anxiety continued to grow as I tossed and turned every night; counting sheep just did not work. I started staying up watching Johnny Carson and other television talk shows in the hopes that they would lull me to sleep. But they seemed to have the reverse effect. I seemed to get a second wind. There were times when the sleepless nights forced me to call in sick to work. I couldn't imagine driving, because when I did drive to work, I felt myself falling asleep in the car. At times, the insomnia was so debilitating, I sometimes pleaded with my husband to drive me in our car around blocks until I fell asleep in the car. As a result of my inability to walk for six weeks because of my back injury, I did not work. My insomnia, the anxiety because of the insomnia, and the depression just escalated. When I did not sleep for four days, my husband took action, and we sought the help of a psychiatrist. I was immediately put on valium to calm me, and an anti-depressant was also prescribed. Unfortunately, while I thought the drugs were assisting me, they were affecting my rationale. I was becoming more and more despondent—and I still had difficulty sleeping.

One of my aunts saw what was happening to me. She suggested I throw away the pills and have a drink—hard liquor—one drink to help me sleep. This sounded like a great idea especially after I had a frightening out-of-body experience when a voice called me to take my life. That evening, I almost did the unthinkable. But out of the blue, something told me to call the head deacon of our church at 3 A.M. When I told him what I wanted to do, when he heard the desperation in my voice, both he and our minister appeared at my door at 4 A.M. to help me. Our minister felt strongly that he had to perform an exorcism on me as I had dabbled in the occult in college and my family used "healers" to cure me of a hernia when I was a child. I allowed the minister to perform this rite, and while I felt lighter after the ritual, that just didn't cure my insomnia. So, I did what my aunt suggested. I threw away all the pills; cold-turkey, I just tossed them down the toilet, not realizing that I should have gradually weaned myself off them. And then I turned to drinking. I must mention that I did not even enjoy alcohol. I liked a glass or two of wine, but hard liquor was not my thing. But it became my thing. And one drink turned into two, or maybe three. But the drinking did not solve my sleepless nights.

I was truly a mess. There were mornings I could not go to work because I had a hangover. I was also diagnosed with a hiatal hernia, reflux, and asthma. I endured walking pneumonia and constant battles with bronchitis and upper respiratory illnesses. And my back still gave me pain from time to time. I was in my mid-thirties, and I felt old. When

I was at my all-time low, one of my former high school students, Will, a wrestler, visited our elementary school in Bedford, NY, at my bequest, where I was the library media specialist. I had loved boxing as a child; my grandfather boxed, and my dad loved watching matches. I was also enamored with wrestling. It was an exciting sport and great entertainment. Will was invited to give a talk about his life and his newfound sport turned career. After his speech, Will visited me in my library. I told him how I was feeling. Obviously, I didn't look great, either. Will told me that I needed to work-out—exercise. I had no desire to do that; although, I did enjoy ballet as a child. I looked at him as if he were crazy. What would I do for a workout? Will asked me to come to his gym as his guest the following week. And I accepted.

I don't know why I accepted. In those days, very few women went to the gym. It was a hang-out for men, a boy's club. I wasn't even sure what to wear, especially since I was overweight. But I went. Embarrassed, I entered the gym where Will warmly greeted me. He took me through an entire work-out. I remember I couldn't even lift five-pound weights. But I sensed that this environment could help me. After the session, he invited me back for several more workouts. I consented.

It was during one of the last sessions with Will that I saw a petite woman working out with very heavy weights. She seemed to be working with a man. I later learned that Sally was a personal trainer, and the man was her client. I had no idea what a personal trainer did for clients, but I carefully observed Sally while she worked with her clientele. She was some motivator; she took clients and molded them—from the inside out. She gave them inspiration, nutritional advice, and pushed them beyond what they thought were their limits.

Gathering up courage one evening, I approached Sally and asked if she and I could talk. We scheduled time for a meeting; and it was during that conversation that I realized Sally had to be my trainer. I had to change. I had to lose weight. I had to get healthier, stronger—not to be perfect—to have a better lifestyle. Sally herself was a natural body builder. She competed and won many body-building contests. I wanted to win, too, at the game of my life. I didn't want to rely on drugs or anything artificial anymore. Sally would be my role model. Sally whipped me into shape over a period. Inhaler in hand, I'd step on the treadmill, do five minutes, step off, inhale two puffs, and get back on. When Sally said, "Do this," I did, even when I doubted that I could. Before long, I was bench pressing twenty-five pounds in each hand; I was using the leg press with three forty-five plates on each side! I did lunges, squats, and shoulder presses. I played outside the gym, rolling tires with Sally and her buddies. I competed with my newfound gym rats. I did what Sally told me because she believed in me like I believed in my students. I made the commitment to show up after work six days a week at Gold's Gym. Sally and I worked together once a week; I followed her written exercise program which she re-wrote as I progressed. I also knew that if I didn't get to the gym right after work, I wouldn't do my work out. I left our daughter in the daycare at Gold's and did my hour or more work out. I met incredibly healthy friends. I sought advice on nutrition, and within a year, lost one dress size. After that year, I made another resolution to eat healthier, and I lost several dress sizes. But the most interesting thing about my exercise routine is what it really did for me; my newly found secret—my workouts gave me confidence.

My secret empowered me. I was stronger than I ever. I also no longer needed my inhaler; I no longer had a hiatal hernia or reflux. I wasn't getting illnesses like bronchitis. I even slept better! I didn't need to drink several drinks to sleep. I didn't need medicines. I was no longer depressed. I went home so happy after exercising that my husband was delighted for me. I felt peaceful even when things around me were difficult. Obstacles didn't seem to matter; I had a different perspective on life, and I was grateful. What a difference from the worn-out young woman listening to demonic messages. But the most powerful thing about my exercise routine is what it secretly did for me.

Much more than a simple barbell weight had been lifted at the gym.

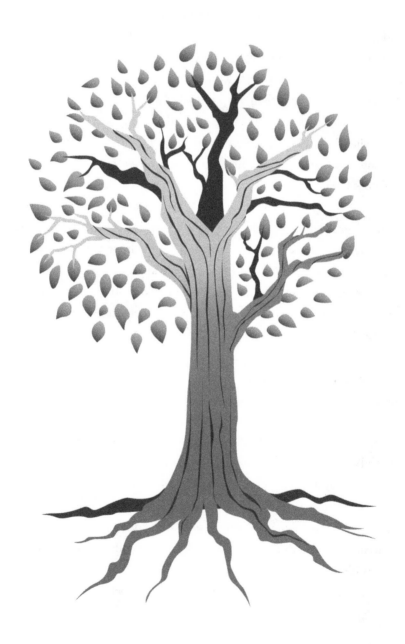

PART IV

THE SAVED BY SPORT RESILIENCY TESTS

CHAPTER 16

THE SAVED BY SPORT RESILIENCY TESTS

INTRODUCTION AND RESOURCES

RESILIENCY NOT ONLY HELPS us cope better with stress, it also allows us to bounce back more quickly from hardship. See how you fair when the going gets tough.

From **http://testyourself.psychtests.com/testid/2121**

How well do you cope? Are you resilient? Do you bounce back from life's trials and tribulations, or do they throw you for a serious loop? Resilience is the quality that allows us to "survive," and even gain strength from hardship. Taking resiliency tests will assess whether you should work on improving your coping skills.

Examine the following statements and indicate which option best describes or applies to you. After finishing this test, you will receive a brief personalized interpretation of your score that includes a graph and information on the test topic I agree to use this test for personal purposes only. Tests available on Psychtests.com are intended for personal use only. Using them for professional purposes constitutes a violation of Psychtest's Terms of Use and will result in suspension of your account.

Here is the link: **http://testyourself.psychtests.com/testid/2121**

HERE ARE TWO ADDITIONAL RESILIENCY QUIZZES FOR YOU TO TAKE:

The Resiliency Quiz by Nan Henderson, M.S.W. (With Permission to Reprint)

https://www.resiliency.com/free-articles-resources/the-resiliency-quiz/

I developed this quiz for anyone—teens, adults, elders—to assess and strengthen the resiliency building conditions in their lives. Use it for yourself or use it as a tool to help others you care about build their resiliency.

PART ONE:

Do you have the conditions in your life that research shows help people to be resilient?

People bounce back from tragedy, trauma, risks, and stress by having the following "protective" conditions in their lives. The more times you answer yes (below), the greater the chances you can bounce back from your life's problems "with more power and more smarts." And doing that is a sure way to increase self-esteem.

Answer yes or no to the following. Celebrate your "yes" answers and decide how you can change your "no" answers to "yes." (You can also answer "sometimes" if that is more accurate than just "yes" or "no".)

1. Caring and Support

_____ I have several people in my life who give me unconditional love, nonjudgmental listening, and who I know are "there for me."

_____ I am involved in a school, work, faith, or other group where I feel cared for and valued.

_____ I treat myself with kindness and compassion and take time to nurture myself (including eating right and getting enough sleep and exercise).

2. High Expectations for Success

_____ I have several people in my life who let me know they believe in my ability to succeed.

_____ I get the message "You can succeed," at my work or school.

_____ I believe in myself most of the time, and generally give myself positive messages about my ability to accomplish my goals–even when I encounter difficulties.

3. Opportunities for Meaningful Participation

_____ My voice (opinion) and choice (what I want) is heard and valued in my close personal relationships.

_____ My opinions and ideas are listened to and respected at my work or school.

_____ I volunteer to help others or a cause in my community, faith organization, or school.

4. Positive Bonds

_____ I am involved in one or more positive after-work or after-school hobbies or activities.

_____ I participate in one or more groups (such as a club, faith community, or sports team) outside of work or school.

_____ I feel "close to" most people at my work or school.

5. Clear and Consistent Boundaries

_____ Most of my relationships with friends and family members have clear, healthy boundaries (which include mutual respect, personal autonomy, and each person in the relationship both giving and receiving).

_____ I experience clear, consistent expectations and rules at my work or in my school.

_____ I set and maintain healthy boundaries for myself by standing up for myself, not letting others take advantage of me, and saying "no" when I need to.

6. Life Skills

_____I have (and use) good listening, honest communication, and healthy conflict resolution skills.

_____I have the training and skills I need to do my job well, or all the skills I need to do well in school.

_____I know how to set a goal and take the steps to achieve it.

PART TWO:

People also successfully overcome life difficulties by drawing upon internal qualities that research has shown are particularly helpful when encountering a crisis, major stressor, or trauma.

The following list can be thought of as a "personal resiliency builder" menu. No one has everything on this list. When "the going gets tough" you probably have three or four of these qualities that you use most naturally and most often. It is helpful to know which are your primary resiliency builders; how have you used them in the past; and how can you use them to overcome the present challenges in your life.

You can also decide to add one or two of these to your "resiliency-builder" menu, if you think they would be useful for you.

PERSONAL RESILIENCY BUILDERS

(Individual Qualities that Facilitate Resiliency)

Put a ✓ by the top three or four resiliency builders you use most often. Ask yourself how you have used these in the past or currently use them. Think of how you can best apply these resiliency builders to current life problems, crises, or stressors.

(Optional) You can then put a + by one or two resiliency builders you think you should add to your personal repertoire.

- ☐ Relationships—Sociability/ability to be a friend/ability to form positive relationships
- ☐ Service—Giving of yourself to help other people; animals; organizations; and/or social causes
- ☐ Humor—Having and using a good sense of humor
- ☐ Inner Direction—Basing choices/decisions on internal evaluation (internal locus of control)
- ☐ Perceptiveness—Insightful understanding of people and situations
- ☐ Independence—"Adaptive" distancing from unhealthy people and situations/autonomy
- ☐ Positive View of Personal Future—Optimism; expecting a positive future
- ☐ Flexibility—Can adjust to change; can bend as necessary to positively cope with situations
- ☐ Love of Learning—Capacity for and connection to learning
- ☐ Self-motivation—Internal initiative and positive motivation from within
- ☐ Competence—Being "good at something"/personal competence
- ☐ Self-Worth—Feelings of self-worth and self-confidence
- ☐ Spirituality—Personal faith in something greater
- ☐ Perseverance—Keeping on despite difficulty; doesn't give up
- ☐ Creativity—Expressing yourself through artistic endeavor, or through other means of creativity

You Can Best Help Yourself or Someone Else Be More Resilient by . . .

1. Communicating the Resiliency Attitude: "What is right with you is more powerful than anything wrong with you."
2. Focusing on the person's strengths more than problems and weaknesses, and asking "How can these strengths be used to

overcome problems?" One way to do this is to help yourself or another identify and best utilize top personal resiliency builders listed in The Resiliency Quiz Part Two.

3. Providing for yourself or others' conditions listed in The Resiliency Quiz Part One.

4. Having patience . . . successfully bouncing back from a significant trauma or crisis takes time.

Note: Here is another mindset quiz online https:// https://neuroheadway. com/wp-content/uploads/2018/09/Resilience-Assessment-Part-1.pdf- what readers will see on the online portal.

RESILIENCY TEST:

1. I often feel like a victim with little or no control over what happens to me.

   - Completely true
   - Mostly true
   - Somewhat true/false
   - Mostly false
   - False

2. What doesn't kill us makes us stronger.

   - Strongly agree
   - Agree
   - Somewhat agree/disagree
   - Disagree
   - Strongly disagree

3. We can overcome painful childhood memories and lessen their influence on our behavior and emotions.

- Strongly agree
- Agree
- Somewhat agree/disagree
- Disagree
- Strongly disagree

4. You hear through the grapevine that one of your friends is hosting a huge birthday bash on the weekend. You rush out and buy a great gift . . . but the invitation never comes! You find yourself at home alone watching reruns on Saturday night. The next Monday everyone is talking about the great party. What's your reaction?

- I feel terribly hurt, but never admit it to anyone. It bothers me for days.
- I am annoyed and demand to know why my friend didn't invite me.
- I am angry and no longer consider him/her a friend.
- I assume it was just a mix-up and forget about it.
- I feel a little hurt and approach my friend and nicely ask why I wasn't invited.
- I feel hurt, but time will heal the wounds.
- I feel hurt but make a joking comment to my friend about it so it doesn't seem like a big deal.
- I feel depressed and think about it for weeks.
- I don't care and don't think about it.

5. You've been working your butt off at work and your boss has finally taken notice. You're sure a promotion is coming any day. When you arrive at the office on a Monday morning, however, you find out that your co-worker got the promotion . . . so you're stuck in the same old grind. How do you react?

- I get angry and confront my boss aggressively; it's not fair!
- I get angry but don't say anything to my boss. It eats away at me for a few weeks.
- I feel frustrated and decide not to get my hopes up anymore, since things never work out.
- I'm very disappointed but feel too uncomfortable to ask my boss about it.
- I'm disappointed but think there must be a reason. I talk to my boss and ask what I need to accomplish to advance.
- I quit my job and lick my wounds for months.
- I don't give it a second thought—all is fair in love and work!

6. When you think about the most difficult times you have faced in the past, what is your first thought?

- "I'm so angry!"
- "I can't think about it without getting physically ill!"
- "Thank God that's behind me!"
- "I wouldn't necessarily want to live it again, but I learned a lot from it."
- "It's some kind of miracle that I survived it; I couldn't do it again."
- "Why do these things happen to me? Life is so unfair!"

7. How would you describe the evolution of your self-esteem over the years?

- It has increased with time and is at the highest it has ever been.
- It's getting worse and worse.
- I've experienced ups and downs, but generally I like myself.
- I don't like myself very much and never have.

8. How strong, overall, do you feel you are emotionally?

- Strong as an ox—I can survive anything.
- I'm usually strong, but I have moments of vulnerability.
- Strong in some ways, vulnerable in others.
- I'm somewhat strong, but I lean more toward vulnerable.
- I'm very vulnerable.
- To be truthful, I can't stand on my own two feet.

9. You arrive at work/school a bit early one morning, and on the way to your office/class you overhear two co-workers/classmates who you don't know very well discussing YOUR character flaws! What do you do?

- I leave it alone; I don't really care what they think.
- I leave it alone; I accept that I cannot possibly please everybody.
- I confront them and tell them that I don't appreciate their behavior.
- I go in the bathroom and let some steam out (by crying/screaming/hitting the wall) but never say anything to them.
- I complain to my supervisor/principal that they are spreading rumors about me.
- I go home and call in sick for the rest of the week.
- I get my revenge by spreading nasty rumors about them.
- I quit school/my job.

10. How long does this event linger in your mind?

- Maximum five minutes
- Less than an hour
- No more than half the day
- All day
- A couple days

TEN WAYS TO BECOME MORE RESILIENT

From https://deepstash.com/article/79478/use-these-10-tips-to-improve-your-resilience

1. Find a sense of purpose.
2. Build positive beliefs in your abilities.
3. Develop a strong social network.
4. Embrace change.
5. Be optimistic.
6. Nurture yourself.
7. Develop your problem-solving skills.
8. Establish goals.
9. Take steps to solve problems.
10. Keep working on your skills.

Identify yourself as a survivor, not a victim.

Ask for help.

RESILIENCY: AN ACRONYM BY
MARILYN GANSEL, PSYD

R—Resources (what are available to me?) Books, Social Network, Environment Change, Libraries etc.

E—Exercise, Movement/Art Therapy

S—Sense of Purpose

I—Include and Embrace Change

L—Learn to Develop and Find Ways to Problem-Solve

I—Include Strategies to Develop Positive Beliefs, Increase Self-Esteem

E—Establish Goals

C—Call On Your Strengths, Nurture Yourself

Y—Yes, I Am a Survivor, Not a Victim

ABOUT THE AUTHORS

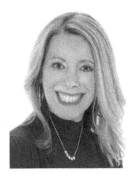

MARILYN GANSEL, AN APPLIED sports psychologist and positive performance coach, helps individuals discover the confidence to stand up, speak out, and take control of their lives. Marilyn's journey has led her to discover the authentic truth about herself, her values, strengths, and inner longings.

She challenges people in every life phase to unleash powerful, destructive thoughts and feelings and take obstacles and turn them into opportunities and possibilities. She expands their thinking and helps them evolve through self-discovery and compassion, thus creating new stories.

This is Marilyn's third book. Her first is *Pain, Purpose, Passion: That Was Then, This Is Now,* twenty-two true stories of triumph through the most challenging times. Her second book is Mac 'N Cheese: Mini Morsels For Positive Performance. Both are available on Amazon.com.

She is available for workshops and seminars as well as one-on-one or group coaching by phone, Zoom, or in person.

www.positiveperformancecoach.org and
marilyn@positiveperformancecoach.org

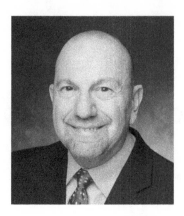

PAUL SCHIENBERG GOT HIS doctorate in clinical psychology from the California School of Professional Psychology in Los Angeles, CA, in 1979. He interned at UCLA/NPI and the Free Foundation. Over the past thirty-five years, he has taught at Redlands University, The New School University, Mount Sinai Medical Center, and The Eastern Group Psychotherapy Society. In addition, he has co-authored a book titled *You Can't Afford to Break Up*. Over the last ten years, Dr. Schienberg has been the publisher and editor of an internet sport psychology magazine called Psyched Online (www.psychedonline.com), featuring interviews with athletes and coaches as well as articles in sport psychology. It is dedicated to helping professional and amateur athletes improve their athletic performance. He meets with athletes directly and teaches sport psychology ideas in a class format. He has a private practice on the Upper East Side of Manhattan, NY.

Dr. Schienberg provides speaking engagements and workshops to amateur and professional athletes who are trying to improve their performance in their sport(s) of choice. In addition, he has had many articles published in nationally known sports magazines.

www.psychedonline.com and
drpaul47@gmail.com

ACKNOWLEDGMENTS

BY MARILYN GANSEL, PsyD

I VIVIDLY REMEMBER MEETING Patricia Horan, editor and publisher of her company, The Roundhouse Press. I was introduced by a client of mine who was also writing a memoir and spoke highly of Patricia. We met in the town of Kent, CT, at a restaurant for lunch.

I was excited to meet her as I wanted her to look at the pages of notes for a book, I was compiling. The stories came from real people I interviewed from all walks of life as an internet radio show host (FTNS). For two years, I met the most incredible people with stories around health, fitness, nutrition, and their ability to overcome major life obstacles. With the interviewee's permission, I took time to speak with each of them to recount their stories of impossible to possible.

Little did I know that Patricia Horan had her own reason for wanting to meet me. She was looking for a life coach who could help her incorporate a healthy, balanced lifestyle in her chaotic world as an author, editor, and publisher. Our friendship began; with it came hours of coaching her and Ms. Horan urging me to write and re-write. And, when it came time for *Saved by Sport*, she initially guided both Paul and me to organize the stories for our title page and to find clever headings for each subdivision. I know she would be proud to see that Paul and I completed our work with the expertise help from Robert Astile. I am forever grateful to her and miss her dearly. Dear Patricia left us too soon in December 2020.

I also want to thank Dick Traum, founder of Achilles International for inspiring physically challenged individuals enjoy athletic events and feel empowered. I thank all the teachers and friends who believed in me when I didn't. Their support in all my endeavors means the world to me. I am also grateful to Joanne and Nan—their books and workshops sharing their insight and wisdom about moving forward, becoming more resilient, and getting in touch with our inner athlete.

ACKNOWLEDGEMENTS
BY PAUL SCHIENBERG, PhD

I AM THANKFUL TO Dick Traum and the Achilles International organization that encourages the physically challenged to participate in athletic events empowering them to lead rich lives.

And, to all who have shared their stories and the stories still to come, you have inspired me and all who meet you in this book. Special thank you to Robert Astle, publisher and editorial director, who created the initial structure and editing of this book. He always provided support and direction when I felt lost and confused. His ability to use the English language added spice to all the stories in the book.

Dick Traum provided inspiration to keep moving forward even when I was not sure how to proceed from story to story and make important commentaries in each. When I would ask for his audience in that regard, he would make himself available to me. In 1983, Dick founded the Achilles Track Club, currently known as Achilles International. He has a BS, MBA, and PhD in Social Psychology from New York University.

We want to give special acknowledgements to all those people who shared their remarkable life stories with us. They became the meat of this book upon which we could comment and share with readers so that they too would be inspired.

Joanne McCaullie, known as Coach P, has been very supportive of our project. She has been a very successful women's college basketball coach at Michigan State University, Maine University, and Duke. She shared very personal information regarding her struggle with bipolar disorder. She has been creating a mental health foundation that is dedicated to removing the shame of having mental struggles and seeking help. In addition, Coach P gave us her ideas and energy in talking through various aspects of our project. Her book, *Secret Warrior*, is an excellent read and contains a much needed perspective for all of us.

Seymore Zelen was the head of my dissertation committee and a great supporter of my becoming a clinical psychologist. His psychology ideas were a great influence on my understanding and approach in the process of helping people with emotional and cognitive problems. He contributed much to attribution theory. I integrated his ideas into the way I thought about people who had suffered traumatic events.

ADDENDUM I

RESEARCH METHODOLOGY

FOR ADDITIONAL REFERENCE, THE authors have provided a methodology on how the interviews were conducted. While this methodology provided the framework and direction for the interviews, other information was given to the authors outside of this format.

METHODOLOGY:

The authors interviewed several individuals and asked extensive questions about their lives, influences, and challenges. They also captured their transformations in terms of their introduction to a life-changing sport. The authors then looked at these interviews, based on what they believed would give the reader the most evocative and powerful experience. The words are 100% from the interviewees, but their stories have been edited for clarity, logic, and repetition.

Here are some of the questions the authors, Dr. Marilyn and Dr. Paul, asked their interviewees:

AGAINST ALL ODDS

1. Describe your early childhood.
2. What was your family like?
3. Were there siblings? How did you interact, communicate?

4. Did you experience rejection? Describe.

5. What were some early struggles related to your illness or disease or life-changing event?

6. Did any significant event in your childhood/adulthood cause or induce the problem?

7. How did you cope with obstacles then? When did this affliction happen—during childhood or later? What event sparked this disorder?

8. How did your family help, or not help?

9. Did any person or other resource help you cope initially during this time?

10. What was school like for you? Was learning difficult or easy?

11. Did you have many friends? Describe your social life?

12. Were you self-confident or did you struggle with your image?

13. What story did you have about yourself that you came to believe, whether it was true or not? How did your story paint how you dealt with hardships?

THE TURNING POINT

1. Who were people who helped you turn your life around?

2. Is there any particular event that helped turn your ship around?

3. Did your thought process change? If so, how?

4. Did your plan come all of a sudden or did it evolve over a period of time?

5. Did you have any idols? If so, who were they and how did they help you change?

6. What was your education?

7. Did you have an occupation, job, or career that you were passionate about or did a career change help you through your process of change and personal growth?

THE PROCESS

1. Looking back on your life, describe your process of change. Were there influential people, a special program, a mental, emotional, or physical change, or awakening that helped you overcome?
2. How did sports, exercise, or your relationship with your body positively transform you? Be specific with stories and examples.
3. What was the greatest and most meaningful experience or event that helped inspire you to deal with your situation?

REWRITING THE STORY

1. How are you now rewriting the story of who you are?
2. Do you feel you are no longer defined by the "old" you? If so, what has shifted for you? What do you want people to know about where you have been and where you are now?
3. How does the mind-body connection affect what decisions you now make about your life?
4. Do you have a mentor? Do you mentor others?

PHYSICAL, SPIRITUAL, & PSYCHOLOGICAL CHANGES

1. Describe your physical, spiritual, and psychological changes? What were they before and what are they now? How have they changed? What had to change for you?
2. Did you engage the help of a psychotherapist? What other professional services did you use to help foster a change? A minister? Alternative healthcare provider? Fitness professional? A class?
3. Did you incorporate mental imagery, visualization, affirmations, hypnosis? What did you find most helpful?

RESILIENCY VERSUS RESIGNATION

1. What gave you the resiliency to bounce back rather than give up?
2. Do you continue to struggle and do you have certain tools in your toolbox that provide the strength to keep on going? If so, what are they?
3. Describe how your sport or exercise keeps you motivated and focused?

PAYING IT FORWARD

1. Now that you have such wisdom in dealing with your situation, how are you helping others?
2. Share success stories.
3. Do you have a team of others who are helping you pay it forward?

ADDENDUM II

UPDATES TO THE STORIES:

JESSE WAS A TWENTY-YEAR-OLD fashion and fitness model in New York City when he woke up on top of a train at Penn Station. Moments later, he was electrocuted, burned alive, and given two days to live.

After surviving 13,800 volts, two months in a coma and thirteen surgeries—including arm amputation, skin grafting, vein re-routing, and bone/muscle/tissue/nerve repair—Jesse has re-learned how to walk, talk, write, and kick ass.

Seven years after doctors deemed him "beyond repair," Jesse, a fitness trainer, model, and motivational speaker in Los Angeles, is inspiring others who are struggling to not just survive—but to thrive.

"There are a lot of people hurting.
Everyone has their pain. Everyone has their story.
But what you think holds you back can actually move you forward."
—Jesse

ADDENDUM III

RESOURCES

THE MINDSET: HERE IS a free online growth mindset test. https://biglifejournal.com/blogs/blog/fixed-mindset-vs-growth-mindset-quiz

Take it and immediately see if you are currently in a fixed or growth mindset.

Dr. Jonice Webb, Your Resource for Relationship & Emotional Health. Emotional Neglect Questionnaire. https://drjonicewebb.com/cen-tips/#.YEYn8iMn12o.mailto

BIBLIOGRAPHY

Bessel, Van der Kolk. *The Body Keeps the Score: Brain, Mind and Body in the Healing of Trauma*. New York: Penguin Books, 2015.

Cordani, David and Traum, Dick. *The Courage to Go Forward*. New York: Morgan James Publishing, 2018.

Currann, Linda. *101 Trauma – Informed Interventions: Activities, Exercises and Assignments to Move the Client and Therapy Forward*. PESI, 2018.

Herman, Judith. *Trauma and Recovery: The Aftermath of Violence*. New York: Basic Books, 1992.

Jackson, Phil and Hugh Delehanty. *Sacred Hoops: Spiritual Lessons of a Hardwood Warrior*. New York: Hachette Books, 1995.

Levine, Peter A. *In an Unspoken Voice: How the Body Releases Trauma and Restores Goodness*. Berkeley: North Atlantic, 2010.

Lancott, Neil, Campy. *The Two Lives of Roy Campanella*. New York: Simon & Schuster, 2011.

Mate, Gabor. *When the Body Says No: I Understand the Stress-Disease Connection*. New York: Random House, 2011.

McCallie, Joanne P. *Secret Warrior: A Coach and Fighter On and Off the Court*. Virginia Beach: Koehler Books, 2021.

Meilli, Trisha. *I am the Central Park Jogger*. New York: Scribner, 2004.

Mumford, George. *The Mindful Athlete: Secrets to Pure Performance.* Berkeley, CA: Parallax Press, 2015.

Pappas, Alexi, *Bravey: Chasing Dreams, Befriending Pain and Other Big Ideas.* New York: Dial Press, 2021.

Traum, Dick and Mike Celizic. *A Victory for Humanity.* Waco, Texas: WRS Publishing, 1993.

Zinn, Jon Kabat and Thich Nat Hanh. *Full Catastrophe Living: Using the Wisdom of Your Body to Face Stress, Pain and Illness, revised edition.* New York, Random House, 2009.

CPSIA information can be obtained
at www.ICGtesting.com
Printed in the USA
LVHW010010040122
707751LV00004B/105